C000078538

POCKET DICTIONARY FOR
NURSES

POCKET DICTIONARY
FOR
NURSES

MARY RALF

ANMOL PUBLICATIONS PVT. LTD.
NEW DELHI - 110 002 (INDIA)

ANMOL PUBLICATIONS PVT. LTD.

4374/4B, Ansari Road, Daryaganj
New Delhi - 110 002
Ph.: 23261597, 23278000
Visit us at: www.anmolpublications.com

Pocket Dictionary for Nurses
© Reserved
First Edition, 1996
Reprint 2004

PRINTED IN INDIA

Published by J.L. Kumar for Anmol Publications Pvt. Ltd.,
New Delhi - 110 002 and Printed at Mehra Offset Press, Delhi.

Preface

Pocket Dictionary for Nurses has been designed to give quick and easy access to a wide range of essential information on all aspects of nursing. The entries are written in a clear explanatory style to provide both straight forward definitions and invaluable background information while an extensive closs-reference system places each entry in a broader scientific context. The entries are arranged in alphabetical order and is based on a systemic reading of medical books and journals published in the 1990s. Cross-references alert you to related words and additional information elsewhere in the dictionary. Approved drug names have been used in the dictionary. A few preparations consisting of a combination of drugs are listed in the dictionary. This dictionary also includes terms on preclinical and paramedical subjects. It is hoped that this dictionary will be an ideal choice for today's nurse.

Mary Ralf

Abdomen. The posterior region of the body trunk of animals. In vertebrates it contains the stomach and intestines and the organs of excretion and reproduction. It is particularly well defined in mammals, being separated from the *thorax by the *diaphragm. In many arthopods, such as insects and spider, it may be segmented.

Abdominal. Pertaining to the abdomen.

Abdominoperineal. Used to describe operation of excision of recturm utilizing approach from both abdominal and perineal incisions.

Abducent nerves. The sixth pair of cranial nerves, activating the external rectus muscle of the eyeball, which rotates the eyeball outwards.

Abduct. Means to draw away from the mid-line.

Abduction. The act of moving a limb away from the middle line of the body.

abductor. Refers to muscle which draws a limb from the meduan line of the body, *e.g.* deltoid.

Ablation. Removal or detachment of a part; or procedure that results in total loss of function of that part.

Ablution. Cleaning by washing.

Abnormal. Irregular, unusual.

Abort. To terminate a process before the full course is run, especially applied to pregnancy.

Abortifacient. A drug taken for the purpose of procuring abortion.

Abortion. Means discharge of the gestation sac from the pregnant uterus before the fetus is viable. Abortion may be *complete* or *incomplete;* it may be *threatened* or *inevitable,* according to the cervical canal being closed or open. Finally it may be *missed* : that is, the fetus may be dead, but may not be discharged immediately. *Tubal A.* When an ovum developing in the Fallopian tube becomes detached, and is thrown off through the abdominal ostium of the tube into the Pouch of Douglas.

Abortus fever. An undulant fever, also called brucellosis, caused by infected cow's milk.

ABO system. One of the most important human *blood group systems. The system is based on the presence or absence of *antigens A and B on the surface of red blood cells and *antibodies against these in blood serum A person whose blood contains either or both these antibodies cannot receive a transfusion of blood containing the corresponding antigens as this would cause the red cells to clump (see agglutination). The table illustrates the basis of the system: people of blood group O are described as 'universal donors' as they can give blood to those of any of the other groups. *See also* immune response.

Group	Antigens on red cell surface	Antibodies in serum	Blood group of people donor can receive blood from	Blood group of people donor can give blood to
A	A	anti-B	A, O	A, AB
B	B	anti-A	B, O	B, AB
AB	A and B	none	A, B, AB, O	AB
O	neither A nor B	anti-A and anti-B	O	A, B, AB, O

The ABO blood group system

Abrasion. A superficial injury to the skin or mucous membrane.

Abreaction. A state of mind brought about during the process of psychoanalysis. The patient lives again through past painful experiences which may unconsciously be causing the neurosis.

Abscess. A collection of pus in a cavity, the result of inflammation. *Alveolar A.* One which develops in the socket of a tooth. *Blind A.* One with no external opening. *Cold A.* One which develops slowly, without inflammation, as in tuberculosis. *Ischiorectal A.* One in the ischiorectal fossa. Metastatic *A.* Secondary to an abscess elsewhere; caused by an infected embolus. *A.* One due to dise ase of the vertebrae. The pus descends in the sheath of the psoas muscle, forming a fluctuating tumour above or below poupart's ligament. It is sometimes tuberculous in origin. *Residual A.* One developing in old inflammatory products. *Stitch A.* One formed around a stitch.

Absolute values. In blood counts these are the actual numbers and not the percentage figures.

Acanthosis. Any disease of the prickle-layer, the lowest stratum of the epidermis. *A. Nigricans.* General pigmentation of the skin with mole-like growths.

Acapnia. A lessened amount of carbon dioxide in the blood often the result of hyperventilation.

Acardia. Congenital absence of the heart.

Acarus. (*ak'-a-rus*), Refers to the name of a group of animal parasites of the spider family, including ticks and mites. A. Scabiei is the parasite causing scabies.

Accessory nevers. Eleventh pair of cranial nerves.

Accidental haemorrhage. Bleeding from the pregnant uterus in the later months of pregnancy due to premature separation of normally situated placenta. It may be *concealed*, when the bleeding remains internal; or external, when the bleeding remains internal; or *external*, when the blood escapes by the vagina.

Accommodation 1. (in animal physiology) The process by which the focal length of the *lens of the eye is changed so that clear. images of objects at a range of distances are displayed on the retina. In man and some other mammals accommodation is achieved by reflex adjustments in the shape of the lens brought about by relaxation and contraction of muscles within the *ciliary body. **2.** (in botany) The ability of a plant to adapt itself to gradually changing enviormental conditions. **3.** (in animal behaviour). The psychological adjustment made by and animal in response to continuously changing environmental conditions.

Accouchement. Childbirth.

Accretion. Accumulation of foreign matter in an organ, *e.g.* the formation of renal calculi.

Acephalic. Headless.

Acetabulum. The cuplike socket in the hip or innominate bone into which the head of the femur fits.

Aceto-acetic acid. Produced at an intermediate stage of fatty acid oxidation. If metabolism is disturbed, as in diabetes mellitus, it is found in excess in the blood and the urine. *Syn*, diacetic acid.

Acetonaemia. The presence of acetone in the blood.

Acetone. A colourless volatile solvent. This substance is formed in the body when metabolism is upset, as in starvation, excessive vomiting, diabetes mellitus. It is excreted in the urine and the breath.

Acetonuria. Means the presence of acetone in the urine.

Acetylcholine. A substance that is released at some (*cholinergic*) nerve endings (*see* neurotransmitter). Its function is to pass on a nerve *impulse to the next nerve (i.e. at a *synapse) or to initiate muscular contraction. Once acetylcholine has been released it has only a transitory effect because it is rapidly broken down by the enzyme *acetylcholinesterase.*

Acetylsalicylic acid. Aspirin.

Achalasia. Failure of relaxation of a muscle sphincter. Applied particularly to the cardiac sphincter, often resulting in dilatation of the oesophagus.

Achilles tendon. The large tendon which attaches the calf muscles to the heel.

Achillorrhaphy. Surgery to rejoin the Achilles tendon after rupture.

Achlorhydria Absence of hydrochloric acid in the gastric juice; may occur in pernicious anaemia and cancer of the stomach.

Acholia. Absence of bile.

Acholuria. The absence of bile pigment from the urine.

Achondroplasia. A form of arrested development of the long bones, leading to dwarfism.

Achromasia. (1) Absence of colour. (2) Loss of staining reaction in a cell.

Achromatopsia. Colour blindness.

Achylia, achylosis. Absence of chyle. *A. gastrica,* atrophy of mucous membrane of the stomach resulting in reduction of absence of gastric juice.

Acidaemia. The blood is abnormally acid and the pH below 7.3.

Acid-base balance. The regulation of the concentrations of acids and bases in blood and other body fluids so that the *pH remains within physiologically acceptable range. This is achieved by the presence of Natural *buffer systems, such as the haemoglobine, Bicarbonate ions, and carbonic acid in mammalian blood. By acting in conjuction, these effectively mop up excess acids and bases and therefore prevent any large shifts in blood pH. The acid-base balance is also influenced by the selective removal of certain ions by the kidneys and the rate of removal of carbon dioxide from the lungs.

Acid-fast. In bacteriology a term applied to certain bacteria which retain the red carbolfuchsin stain after the application of an acid solution. Other organisms are decolorized.

Tubercle and leprosy bacilli are 'acid-fast'.

Acidosis. A condition in which the acid-base balance of the body fluids is disturbed, resulting in a fall in pH.

Acid phosphatase. Enzyme produced by the prostate gland and secreted in seminal fluid. Serum acid phosphatase is raised in carcinoma of the prostate when there is bone involvement.

Acinus. A minute grape-like structure whose cells secrete; as in the breast. Acini are also found in the lungs and other racemose glands. Syn. alveolus, pl. alveoli.

Acne. Inflammation of the sebaceous glands of the skin, causing the formation of little pustules, and of blackheads. Often found among adolescents.

Acousma. The hearing of imaginary sounds.

Acquired characteristics. Features that are developed during the lifetime of an individual e.g. the enlarged arm muscles of a tennis player. It is a basic tenet of current evolutionary thought that such characteristics are not genetically controlled and cannot be passed on to the next generation. *See also* Lamarckism; neo-Lamarckism.

Acrocephaly. Congenitally malformed cone-shaped head.

Acrocyanosis. Blueness of the extremities.

Acromegaly. A disease marked by enlargement of the face, hands and feet, and due to a pathological condition of the pituitary gland. The commonest form of gigantism.

Acromion. The outward projection of the spine of the scapula.

Acronyx. Means an ingrowing of the nail.

Acroparaesthesia. The term used for a tingling feeling in the hands with numbness caused by pressure on the brachial plexus.

Acrophobia, Morbid fear of being at a height.

ACTH (adrenocorticotrophic hormone, corticotrophin).
A hormone produced by the anterior *pituitary gland in
response to stress that controls secretion of certain hormones (the *corticosteroids) by the adrenal glands. It can
be administered by injection to treat such disorders as
rheumatic diseases and asthma, but it only relieves
symptoms and is not a cure.

Actinodermatitis. Inflammation of the skin from ultra-violet
or other rays.

actinomyces. A pathogenic fungus causing actinomycosis.

Actinomycosis. Disease due to Actinomyces. There are
usually chronic discharging abscesses.

Actinotherapy. Treatment by ultraviolet and infra-red radia-
tions.

Action potential. The chage in electrical potential that occurs across a cell membrane during the passage of a
nerve *impulse. As an impulse travels in a wavelike
manner along the *axon of a nerve, it causes a localized
and transient switch in electrical potential across the cell
membrane from -60 mV (millivolts) to + 45 mV. Nervous stimulation of a muscle fibre has a similar effect.

Action tremor. Tremor of limbs or incoordination of movement as in ataxia.

Active movements. A term used by physiotherapists to
denote normal movement of a limb or part of the body.

Active principle. The substance in a drug which gives it a
medicinal character.

Acupuncture. (1) A treatment to relive oedema. The
oedematous tissue—usually of the legs—is stabbed all
over with straight cutting needles. (2) A from of general
treatment given by those who practise, 'fringe' medicine.

Acute. Rapid; severe *A. abdomen.* A surgical emergency resulting from disease or damage of abdominal viscera.

Acute yellow atrophy. Severe damage to liver due to toxic agent.

Acystia. Absence of bladder.

Adam's apple. The laryngeal prominence formed by the thyroid cartilage.

Adamantinoma. Epitheliat tumour of jaw.

Adaptation. 1. Any change in the structure or functioning of an organism that makes it better suited to its environment. *Natural selection of inheritable adaptations ultimately leads to the development of new species. Increasing adaptation of a species to a particular environment tends to diminish its ability to adapt to any sudden change in that environment. 2. The alteration in the degree of, sensitivity (either an increase or a decrease) of a sense organ to suit conditions more extreme than normally enountered. An example is the adjustment of the eye to vision in very bright or very dim light.

Addiction. State of physical and mental dependence on a drug, usually alcohol or narcotics.

Addis count. Number of red blood cells in the urine, per 24 hours.

Addison's anaemia. Pernicious anaemia.

Addison's disease. A disease A the suprarenal gland causing anaemia, vomiting, wasting, low blood pressure and bronzed skin.

Adducent muscle of eye. Internal rectus muscle.

Adduct. To draw towards the midline.

Adduction. The act of moving a limb towards the midline of the body.

Adductor. A muscle which draws towards the midline of the body, e.g. *A. muscles* of the thigh draw the legs together.

Adendritic. A nerve cell without dendrons.

Adenectomy. Excision of a gland.

Adenine. *purine derivative. It is one of the major component bases of nucleotides and the nucleic acids *DNA and *RNA.

Adenitis. Inflamation of a gland.

Adenocarcinoma. A carcinomatous tumour of a gland.

Adenoid. Lymphoid tissue, in the nasopharynx, which when swollen hinders breathing.

Adenoidectomy. Operation to remove adenoids.

Adenoma. A benign tumour of glandular tissue.

Adenomyoma. A benign growth, esp. in uterus, of glandular and muscle tissue.

Adenopathy. A disease of a gland, especially a lymphatic gland.

Adenovirus. One of a group of DNA-containing viruses found in rodents, fowl, cattle, monkeys, and man. In man they produce acute respiratory-tract infections with symptoms resembling those of the common (see oncogenic) cold. They are also implicated in the formation of tumours (see oncogenic).

Adermin. Pyridoxin of vitamin B6, concerned with the metabolism of amino-acids.

Adiaphoresis. Deficiency of perspiration.

Aditus. An entrance. A portal. *A. and antrum* is the narrow passage between the mastoid antrum and the tympanic cavity of the ear.

Adjuvant. A secondary ingredient in a prescription, aiding the chief drug.

Adnexa. Appendages. Usually applied to the uterine appendages.

Adolescence. The period between puberty and maturity.

Adrenal glands. A pair of endocrine glands situated immediately above the kidneys (hence they are also known as the *suprarenal glands*) The inner portion of the adrenals, the *medulla*, secretes the hormones *adrenaline and *noradrenaline; the outer *cortex* secrets small amounts of sex hormones (*androgens and *oestrogens) and various *corticosteroids, which have a wide range of effects on the body. *See also* ACTH.

Adrenalectomy. The removal of one or both adrenal glands.

Adrenaline (epinephrine). A hormone, produced by the medulla of the *adrenal glands, that increases heart activity, improves the power and prolongs the action of muscles, and increases the rate and depth of breathing to prepare the body for 'fright, flight, or fight', At the same time it ihbibits digestion and excretion. Similar effects are produced by stimulation of the *sympathetic nervous system. Adrenaline can be administered by injection to relieve bronchial asthma and reduce blood loss during surgery by constricting blood vessels.

Adrenergic. Describing a nerve fibre that either release *adrenaline or *noradrenaline when stimulated or is itself stimulated by these substances. *Compare* cholinergic.

Adrenocortical steroids. Endocrine secretions of the adrenal cortex.

Adrenogenital syndrome. Development of secondary male characteristics in the female or secondary female characteristics in the male. Usually due to hyperplasia or adenoma of the adrenal cortex.

Adrenolytic. A drug antagonistic to adrenaline.

Adrenotropin, Also called adrenocorticotrophic hormone. An anterior pituitary hormone acting upon the adrenal gland.

Adulteration. Fraudulent addition of unnecessary substances to foods or medicines.

Advancement. An operation for the cure of squint. The procedure consists in dividing one of the eye muscles at its insertion into the eyeball and reattaching it farther forward.

Adventitia. Outer coat of a blood vesel.

Aedes aegypti. Species of mosquito transmitting yellow fever, etc.

Aerobes. Term applied to bacteria needing oxygen for respiration, cf, anaerobes.

Aerobic. Requiring free oxygen or air to support life.

Aerocele. A diverticulum of larynx, trachea or bronchus.

Aerogen. Any gasproducing bacterium, *e.g. Clostridium welchii*, the cause of gas gangrene.

Aerophagy. Excessive air swallowing.

Aetiology. The science of the causation of disease.

Afebrile. Without fever.

Affective disorders. Group of psychiatricillnesses primarily due to reaction to internal or external stress. They include anxiety states, depression, mania and hypomania.

Afferent. Carrying from the outer regions of a body or organ towards its centre. The term is usually applied two types of nerve fibres or blood vessels. *Compare* efferent.

Affiliation. The fixing of paternity of an illegitimate child on the putative father.

Afterbirth. The *placenta, *umbilical cor and *extraembryonic membranes, which are expelled from the womb after a mammalian fetus is born. In most non-human mammals the afterbirth, which contains, nutrients and might otherwise attract predators, is eaten by the female.

After-image. A retinal impression persisting although the stimulus of light has eased.

After-pains. Pains from uterine contractions following labour.

Agammaglobulinaemia. Absence of deficiency of gamma globulin in plasma proteins, leading to inadequate response to infection.

Agar. An extract of certain species of red seaweeds that is used as a gelling agent in mecrobiological *culture media, foodstuffs, medicines, and cosmetic creams and jellies. *Nutrient agar* consists of a broth made from beef extract or blood that is gelled with agar and used for the cultivation of bacteria, fungi, and some algae.

Agglutination. The clumping together by antibodies of microscopic foreign particles (*antigens), such as red blood cells or bacteria, so that they form a visible pellet-like precipitate. Agglutination is a specific reaction, *i.e.* a particular antigen will only clump in the presence of its specific antibody; it therefore provides a means of identifying unknown bacteria and determining *blood group. When red cells of incompatible blood groups (e.g. group A and group B - *see* ABO system) are mixed together agglutination of the cells occurs (haemagglurination).

Agglutinins. Antibodies such as those found in the blood serum of persons suffering from typhoid or paratyphoid fever. They have the property of causing bacteria to clump together or 'agglutinate'.

Agglutinogen. A factor stimulating the production of specific antibodies in the blood.

Aglutition. Inability to swallow.

Agonist. Muscle which shortens when in action.

Agoraphobia. Neurotic fear of open spaces.

Agranulocyte. The non-granular leucocytes *i.e.* monocytes and lymphocytes.

Agranulocytosis. Absence or marked reduction in the blood of the polymorphonuclear cells. May be caused by drugs such as the sulphonamides or irradiation of the bone maroow.

Agraphia. Means loss of the power to express words and ideas in writing.

Ague. *See* Malaria.

AID. Artificial insemination (donor other than husband).

AIH. Artificial insemination with semen from the husband.

Air. *See* Atomosphere *A.*, *tidal.* The air breathed in and out in ordinary breathing.

Air embolism. Embolism caused by air entering the circulatory system.

Air-encephalography. Radiography of the brain after air has been introduced into the subarachnoid space.

Air hunger. Respiratory distress caused by lack of available oxygen especially in haemorrhage.

Akinesis. Loss or imperfection of movement.

Al. Chemical symbol for aluminium.

Ala. A wing, *A nasi.* The outer side of the external nostril.

Alastrim. Variola minor.

Albee's operation. (1) The hip joint is ankylosed by a plastic operation. (2) A bone grafting operation to the spine performed in tuberculous disease of the spine. The graft is taken from the tibia.

Albers-Schönberg's disease. Marble bone disease.

Albino. A male with white hair, fair skin, and pink eyes, due to pigmentary deficiency.

Albumin. Serum protein with relatively low molecular weight (MW = 70,000) which is of great importance in

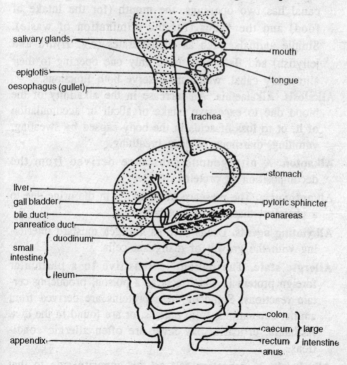

The human alimentary canal

Labels: salivary glands, mouth, epiglotis, tongue, oesophagus (gullet), trachea, liver, stomach, gall bladder, pyloric sphincter, bile duct, panareas, panreatice duct, small intestine { duodinum, ileum }, colon, caecum, rectum, large intenstine, appendix, anus controlling water exchanges between the blood and tissue fluids.

Albuminuria. Albumin in the urine; occurs in diseases of the kidneys. Nowadays known as proteinuria.

Alimentary canal. A tubular organ in animals that is divided into a series of zones specialized for the ingestion, *digestion, and *absorption of food and for the elimination of indigestible material. In most animals the canal has two openings, the mouth (for the intake of food) and the *anus (for the elimination of waste). Simple animals, such as coelenterates (*e.g. Hydra* and jellyfish) and flatworms, have only one opening to their alimentary canal, which must serve both functions.

Alkalosis. Alkalaemia. An increase in the alkalinity of the blood due to excessive intake of alkali or accumulation of it, or to loss of acids in the body caused by sweating, vomiting, diarrhoea or deep breathing.

Alkapton. A nitrogenous substance derived from the decomposition of proteins.

Alkaptonuria. The presence of alkaption in the urine due to a chemical disorder of metabolism.

Alkylating agents. Drugs such as nitrogen mustard interfering with the growth of malignant cells.

Allergic state. The patient is sensitive to a particular foreign protein is which acts as a poison, producing certain reactions. Some of these proteins are derived from animal emanations, from pollens, or are found in the diet. Asthama, urticaria, hay fever are often allergic conditions.

Allocheiria. A sensation felt on the opposite side to that which is touched.

Allograft. Graft with material obtained from a donor.

Alveoli. (Sing. is alveolus.) (1) The sockets of the teeth. (2) The air cells in the lungs. (3) The secreting units of the breasts.

Alveolitis. Inflammation of an alveolus.

Alzheimer's disease. Degeneration of the brain cortex. Loss of memory, aphasia, and paralysis occur.

Amastia. Absence of breasts.

Amaurosis. Blindness from disease or defect of the nervous system of the eye; occurs in uraemia.

Amaurotic Family idiocy. This condition, also known as Tay-Sach's disease, occurs in infants. There is optic atrophy, rigidity of the limbs and coma.

Amentia. Absence of intellect; idiocy.

Ametria. Absence of uterus.

Ametropia. Defective vision due to abnormal form or refractive power of the eye.

Amino-acids. Nitrogen-containing organic acids of which proteins are built. Ten are considered to be essential to health and must be present in the food. They are leucine, phenylalanine, lysine, arginine, histidine, valine, tryptophane, isoleucine, methionine and threonine.

Aminopterin. A folic acid antagonist.

Amnesia. Loss of memory. *Anterograde A.* Inability to remember recent events. *Retrograde A.* Symptom of concussion. The patient cannot remember what happened immediately before the accident.

Amniocentesis. Aspiration of liquor amnii from the uterus for diagnostic purposes.

Amniography. Radiographic demonstration of amniotic sac by injection of radio-opaque dye.

Amoeba. A microscopic unicellular animal, one variety of which causes amoebic dysentery.

Amoebiasis. Infection with pathogenic amoebae (plural of amoeba).

Amoebicide. Substance lethal to amoeba.

Amphiarthrosis. A slightly movable joint, *e.g.* the articulations of the spine.

Ampoule. A sealed phial containing some drug or solution sterilized ready for use.

Ampulla. Any flask-shaped dilatation. A. of vater.

Amputation. The removal of a limb or organ.

Amylase. An enzyme which has a digestive action on carbohydrates. It converts starch into maltose. It is found as ptyalin in the saliva and as amylopsin in the pancreas.

Amyloid disease. also called fatty or lardaceous disease. Wax-like material is laid down in the liver, kidneys, spleen and blood vessels. It usually occurs as a result of long-standing infection.

Amyotonia. A form of muscular feebleness or paralysis, often congenital.

Anabolic compound. Chemical substance which helps to repair body tissue.

Anacrotism. A small additional wave or notch found in the ascending limb of the tracing of the pulse curve.

Anaemia. Diminished oxygen-carrying capacity of the blood, due to a reduction in the number of red cells or in their content of haemoglobin, or both. The cause may be inadequate production of red cells or excessive loss of blood. (For different types, *e.g.* Pernicious A., See under special name.) See Blood count.

Anaerobe. Any micro-organism that can live and multiply in the absence of free oxygen, *e.g.* tetanus.

Anaesthesia. Absence of sensation; loss of feeling *Basal A.*

Partial general anaesthesia obtained by a drug such as morphine given before an inhalation anaesthesia. *Dissociated A.* Loss of sensation to pain and temperature, sense of touch being retained. *General A.* This gives loss of consciousness. *Glove A.* Hysterical loss of feeling in the area of the hand a glove covers. *Intravenous A.* A General anaesthesia produced by intravenous injection. *Local A.* Anaesthesia of a certain area only. *Nerve block A.* Local anaesthesia produced by injecting an anaesthetic into a sensory nerve. *Rectal A.* General anaesthesia by administering an anaesthetic rectally. *Refrigeration A.* Anaesthesia produced by intense cold. *Spinal A.* An anaesthetic is injected into the subarachnoid space of the spinal cord producing anaesthesia in the lower half of the body.

Anaesthetic. An agent which produces insensibility. (As an adjective it means insensible to touch.)

Anaesthetist. The administrator of anaesthetics.

Analeptic. A restorative. A drug which restores to consciousness, *e.g.* nikethamide.

Analgesia. Diminished sensibility to pain. A symptom in certain nervous diseases, *e.g.* syringomyelia.

Analgesic. relieving pain; remedy for pain.

Anastomosis. In anatomy the intercommuincation of the terminal branches of two or more blood vessels. In surgery the establishment of some artificial connection, as, for instance, between two parts, of the intestine.

Anatomy. The science of organic structure. *A., applied.* As applied to diagnosis and treatment.

Aneurysm needle. A blunt instrument which can be passed under a vessel; the eye is then threaded and the needle withdrawn, leaving the ligature beneath the vessel ready to tie.

Angina pectoris. A disease characterized by sense of suffocation, with pain in the chest due to insufficient blood supply to the heart, the arteries being diseased. It occurs on effort. Sublingual glyceryl trinitrate is helpful.

Angiosarcoma. A sarcoma composed of vascular tissue.

Angiospasm. The blood vessels contract in spasms.

Angiotensin. A polypeptide raising blood pressure and formed by the action of renin on plasma globulins.

Ankle. The joint between the leg and the foot. The bones which articulate are the tibia and fibula above and the talus below.

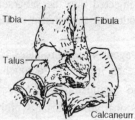

The ankle joint

Ankylosing spondylitis. Disease of joints, of unknown aetiology, in which destruction of the joint space occurs and is followed by sclerosis and calcification. The sacroiliac joints are predominantly affected.

Ankylosis. Immobility in a joint, following inflammation or prolonged immobilization. *False A.* Fixation or stiffness produced by conditions around the joint, such as contraction of skin, *e.g.* after burns, or of tendons, by ossification of muscles, or by outgrowths of bone. *True A.* Fixation or stiffness produced by conditions in the joint such as injury or arthritis. *Fibrous A.* Fixation by fibrous tissue. *Bony A.* the articular surfaces of the bones are fused together.

Anopheles. A genus of mosquitoes. They are carriers of the malarial parasite, their bite being the means of transmitting the disease to human beings.

Anorchous. Having no testes, or the condition in which the testes have not descended into the scrotum.

Anteflexion. A bending forward, as of the normal position of the uterus.

Ante mortem. Before death.

Anteversion. The state of being inclined forword. It is the normal position of the uterus.

Anthelmintic. A remedy for intestinal worms *e.g.* santonin, extract of filixv mas, etc.

Anthracosis. Disease caused by inhaling coal dust or soot into the lungs. Seen in miners.

Anthrax. An acute, infectious disease produced by the Anthrax bacillus. *Skin A.* and *Pulmonary A.* and the two main forms.

Anthropoid, Manlike. *A apes* include animals most closely related to man. *A pelvis* has a narrowed transverse inlet which is long antero-posteriorly.

Anthropology. The natural history of mankind.

Anti. Prefix meaning against.

Antibiotic. Opposed to life; drugs used in the treatment of bacterial infections.

Antibodies. Protein substances, usually circulating in the blood, which neutralize corresponding antigens.

Anticholinergic. Term applied to drugs inhibiting the action of acetylcholine.

Anticoagulant. Substance which delays the clotting of blood.

Anticonvulsant. A drug used to prevent a convulsion.

Antidepressants. Drugs used to treat depression. They may be mono- amine oxidase inhibitors, or the imipramine group of drugs.

Antidiuretic hormone. Posterior pituitary hormone regulating the amount of water passing from the uriniferous tubules into the renal substance.

Antidote. The corrective to a poison.

Antigen. Substance capable of stimulating the formation of antibodies.

Antihistamine. Drug counteracting the effects of the liberation of histamine in the tissues, *e.g.* Anthisan, Benadryl, Dramamine, Phenergan, etc.

Anti-infective factor. Found in vitamin A.

Antimetabolites. Chemical substances used to prevent cell division in malignant disease.

Antimitotic. Substance which prevents mitosis.

Antispasmodic. An agent relieving spasm.

Antistatic. Preventing a build-up of static electricity.

Antithrombin. A substance in the blood having the power of retarding or preventing coagulation.

Antithyroid drugs. Substances which restrict the secretion of thyroid hormones by interference in the intermediary metabolism of the gland.

Antitoxin. A specific antibody produced in the blood in response to a toxin or poison. The antibody is capable of neutralizing that particular toxin.

Antitragus. The prominence of the lower portion of the external ear.

Antivenin. An antidote injected in cases of poisoning by snake bite.

Antrostomy. Incision of an antrum.

Antrum. A cave; applied to the maxillary sinus, called the antrum of Hinghmore, and the cavity in the mastoid bone communicating with the middle ear.

Anuria. Cessation of the production of urine; to be distinguished from retention of urine, due to inability to empty the bladder.

Anus, The rectal exit. *Imperforate A.* A congenital malformation where a child is born with no anal opening, or an anus is present but does not communicate with the bowel above. Treatment is operative and success depends on degree of development of lower bowel.

Anxiety neurosis. A neurosis in which fear and apprehension mainly control the patient's behaviour and ideas.

Aorta. The large artery arising from the left ventricle of the heart and supplying blood to the whole body.

Aortic incompetence. Blood from the aorta regurgitates back into the left ventricle, due to inefficiency of the valve.

Aortic stenosis. Narrowing of the aortic valve due to malformation or disease.

Aortic valves. Three semi-lunar valves guarding the entrance from the left ventricle to the aorta and preventing the backward flow of the blood.

Aortitis. Inflammation of the aorta.

Apathy. Listlessness. Lack of activity.

Apepsia. Failure of digestion due to deficiency of gastric juice.

Aperient. A purgative medicine, *e.g.* cascara.

Aperistalsis. Cessation of peristalsis.

Apex. Top, extreme point, summit. *A. of the heart.* Narrow

end of heart enclosing left ventricle. *A. beat.* The heart
beat as felt at its most forcible point on the chest wall.
This corresponds with the position of the apex of the left
ventricle.

Apgar score. System for assessing vitality of new-born infant, esp. heart rate and respiratory effort.

Aphagia. Inability to swallow.

Aphakia. Absence of lens of the eye.

Aphasia. Speechlessness; due to disease or injury of brain.

Aphonia. Loss of voice.

Appendices epiploicae. Small peritoneal bags of fat projecting from the peritoneal coat of the large intestine.

Appendicitis. Inflammation of the appendix.

Appendix vermiformis. A wormlike offshoot from the
caecum, ending blindly, and 1 to 5 in long.

Apperception. The conscious reception a sensory impression.

Areola. The pigmented skin round the nipple of the breast.

Areolar tissue. Filmy connective tissue of the body.

Argentaffinoma. Also known as carcinoid tumour. Arises

Areola of breast: A = Nipple
B = Montgomery's tubules
C = Primary areola
*D = Secondary areola, develops in the early weeks of preg-
nancy.*

from so-called argentaffin cells in the gastro-intestinal tract.

Arginine. One of the essential amnio-acids formed from the digestion of dietary protein. It is present as a stage in urea formation.

Artefact. A lesion produced by artificial means.

Arterial. Pertaining to an artery. Thus arterial tension means the pressure of the blood circulating in a given artery.

Arteriectomy. Excision of part of an artery.

Arteriography. To demonstrate blood vessels following the injection of contrast medium opaque to x-rays.

Arterioles. Small arteries with contractile muscular walls which control the supply of blood to the capillaries.

Arteriopathy. Disease of the arteries.

Arterioplasty. Surgery to reform and artery, especially for aneurysm.

Arteriorrhaphy. Of an artery.

Arterio-sclerosi. Degeneration of an artery with hardening of its walls, seen chiefly in old age. The condition is accompanied by high blood pressure.

Arteriotomy. Incising an artery.

Arthrography. Radiography of joint after the injection of radio- opaque fluid to outline the joint space.

Arthropathy. Disease of the joints. Commonly used to imply secondary damage to joints as a result of other disease processes.

Arthroplasty. The making of an artificial joint.

Arthrotomy. Incision into a joint.

Articular. Relating to the joints; the articulation of a skeleton is the manner in which the bones are joined together.

Articulation, (1) A joint between two or more bones. (2)

The enunciation of words.

Artificial feeding, Feeding of an infant with food other than its mother's milk.

Artificial insemination, Artificial introduction of spermatozoa into the vagina.

Artificial kidney. Dialysing apparatus through which blood from the patient is pumped so that excretory products such as urea may be extracted in the event of the patient's own kidneys not functioning.

Aschoff nodules. The focal lesions of acute rheumatism consisting of perivascular necrosis of collagen. These nodules tend to occur in the heart, muscles and connective tissues.

Aseptic. Free from pathogenic micro-organisms. In aseptic surgery, all instruments, dressings, etc., are sterilized before use.

Asexual. Having no sex. A method of reproduction in which there is no gamete formation.

Astigmatism. Inequality in the curvature of the cornea or lens, with consequent blurring and distortion of the images thrown upon the retina.

Atavism. The recurrence of some hereditary peculiarity which has skipped one or more generations.

Athetosis. A condition marked by continuous and purpose-less movements, especially of the hands and fingers.

Athlete's heart. Aortic incomperhence from strain. *A. foot.* Infectious disease of the skin between and behind the toes, due to parasitic fungi.

Atlas. First cervical vertebra.

Atrio-ventricular bundle. A neuromuscular bundle of fibres connecting the atria with the ventricles of the heart, by means of which the impulse to contract is conducted. Degeneration of this bundle produces heart-block, a condition in which the ventricle contracts independently of the atrium.

Atrophy. Wasting of a part, from disuse or lack of nutrition.

Atropine. The active principle of belladonna. It paralyses parasympathetic nerve endings, therefore inhibits glandular secretions, and peristalsis, increases the rate of the heart beat and dilates the pupil of the eye. It is used to inhibit bronchial secretion before and anaesthetic and 0.6mg atropine sulphate may be given subcutaneously together with 15mg morphine sulphate. To dilate the pupil of the eye, drops are instilled in a 1 per cent solution.

Auerbach's plexus. The collection of nerve fibres (terminations of vagus and sympathetic nerves) and ganglia situated in the intestinal wall. Function: regulates peristalsis.

Auto-infection. Self-infection.

Auto-intoxication. Poisoning by toxins generated within the body.

Autolysis. The process of self-digestion occurring in tissues under pathological condition and in the uterus during the puerperium.

Automatism. A condition in which actions are performed without consciousness or regulated purpose; sometimes follows a major or minor epileptic fit.

Autonomic nervous system. Motor supply to smooth muscle and glands. Divided into sympathetic and parasympathetic systems and characterized by synapsing in ganglia after fibres leave the central nervous system. Not directly under conscious control but there is considerable cortical representation.

Auto-radiography. Photography showing localization of radioactive substance in a tissue section.

Axon. The long process of nerve cell conducting impulses away from the cell body.

Axonotmesis. Damage causing the break-up of nerve fibres but the supporting tissue remains intact.

Azoospermia. Absence of viable sperms in the semen causing male sterility.

Azotaemia. Excess urea in the blood.

Azoturia. An increase of urea in the urine.

Azygos. Not paired but single.

B

Babinski's reflex. Extensor plantar reflex. Extension instead of flexion of the great toe on stroking the sole of the foot. The sign is normal in infants and abnormal after about two years.

Bacillary dysentery. Infection of the gut with Shigella bacilli.

Bacilluria. Bacilli in the urine.

Bacitracin. Antibiotic from the Bacillus subtilis group. Sometimes used externally to treat skin infections.

Bacteraemia. Bacteria in the blood.

Bacteria. Microscopic unicellular living organisms; some cause disease and are called pathogenic. The principal forms are: (1) *Cocci*, those which are rounded in shape. When these are disposed in pairs they are called *Diplococci*— these occur in- pneumonia, some forms of meningitis, and gonorrhoea. When these occur in chains they are called *Streptococci*, when in clusters *Staphylococci*. (2) *Bacilli* are rod-shaped bacteria which include the Gram-positive organisms causing anthrox, tetanus and diphtheria; Gram-negative causing dysentery, typhoid and plague and the acid-fast organisms of tuberculosis and leprosy. (3) *Spirilla* are corkscrew-like germs, or spiral rods with several twists, occurring in relapsing fever, and syphilis. The majority of bacteria are stationary, but some have power of movement. Bacteria have power of multiplying by splitting across their centre, this is known as binary fission: others form spores, which are small, round, glistening bodies able to withstand great extremes of heat and cold.

Bacteriophage. Micro-organism, resembling a virus, capable of attacking other larger micro-organism and destroying them by lysis.

Bacteriostatic. Preventing the growth of bacteria.

Bacteriuria. Bacteria in the urine.

Bainbridge reflex. Increased venous return causing increased heart rate and thought to be associated with inhibition of vagal impulses.

Bandage. An appliance, generally of woven material, used to give support, apply pressure or secure a dressing.

Baroreceptor nerves. Found in the carotids and arch of the aorta. They stem from the vagus and glossopharyngeal nerves.

Brrier nursing. The nursing of a patient with an infectious disease in a general ward, or a ward with patients having a variety of infectious diseases. Adequate precautions are taken so that cross infection does not occur.

Bartholin's glands. Two small glands, one each side of the vulva, may develop into an abscess or its duct may distend into a cyst.

Basal metabolism. The amount of energy consumed in essential physiological processes without taking into account any voluntary activity.

Basal narcosis. Sleep produced by drugs given before an anaesthetic.

Bath. Any liquid or gas used to bath the body. A *waterb.* may be cold, 32-70° F (0-21°C) used to stimulate body tissues; a warm bath is 90-104° F (32-40°C) and a hot bath is 98-108 0F (37-42 °C) and may be analgesic, sedative and diaphoretic. *Medicated bs.* These may contain sodium bicarbonate, saline, wax, *etc.* Starch, oatmeal and bran were formerly much used for emollient purposes.

Bassini's. herniorrhophy Method of reconstruction of the inguinal canal in repair of hernia.

Battered baby. A young child physically injured by his parent or his guardian. *B.b* syndrome. A recognized pattern of physical maltreatment of a young child by his parents. The parents are themselves psychologically disordered.

Bedsore. A sore on the buttocks, heels, ankles, shoulders or elbows, caused by constant pressure on these points when lying. This may arise in long illnesses if pressure is not relived, and is specially likely to occur in cases of spinal injury if the patient is not frequently turned. Now usually called pressure sore.

Benedict's solution. May be used in testing urine for sugar.

Benign. Non-malignant. Non cancerous.

Bennett's fracture. Fracture of the base of the first metacarpal due to a blow on the base of the thumb.

Biceps. The two-headed muscle in front of the humerus.

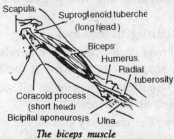

The biceps muscle

Bicuspid. Having two points or cusps. The two teeth immediately behind the canines in each jaw are bicuspids. Becuspid or mitral valve, the valve between the left atrium and left ventricle of the heart.

Bielchowski's disease. Early juvenile cerebro-macular degeneration, characterized by mental deterioration and blindness.

Bile. Gall. The secretion of the liver; greenish, bitter, and viscid. Alkaline. Specific gravity 1010 to 1040. It consists of water, inorganic salts, bile salts, bile pigments. It emulsifies fats and stimulates peristalsis.

Bile pigments. Bilirubin, red, and biliverdin, green. These pigments are derived from haemoglobin and appear in the faces as stercobilin, and in the urine as urobilin. In cases of jaundice the unaltered pigments bilirubin and biliverdin appear in the urine.

Bilharzia. The same as Schistosoma. A parasitic worm infesting the portal vein and lymph spaces. The worm's eggs are the main cause of the symptoms in those affected; they are spiny, and therefore cause bleeding wherever they lodge. They are found in enormous numbers in the bladder and rectum.

Biniodide of mercury. A very poisonous antiseptic, similar in composition and properties to perchloride of mercury, but less irritating and less potent. *See* corrosive sublimate.

Binocular. Relating to both eyes.

Binovular. Produced by two ova. Binovular twins develop from two separate ova fertilized at the same time.

Bio-assay. Quantitative estimation of bilogically active substances such as hormones.

Biochemistry. The chemistry of cell life.

Biogenesis. Hypothesis that living matter always arises from living matter.

Biology. The science of life and living organisms.

Biopsy. Examination of tissue from the living body.

Bios. The Greek word for life; hence the derivation of such words as 'biology', 'biogenesis'.

Biot's respiration. Seen most commonly in menigitis. There are pauses in the respiration, but no waxing or waning as in Cheyne- Stokes respiration.

Biparous. Bearing twins.

Birth. The act of being born. *B.* mark, congenital naevus. *B.* paralysis, paralysis due to injury at birth.

Black stools. Sign of bleeding from the intestine. May also occur in patients taking large quantities of iron tablets.

Blackwater fever. A form of malaria in which there is rapid haemolysis of red blood cells so that the blood supply to vital organs such as the brain is impaired. There is high fever, haemoglobinuria and jaundice.

Bladder. A hollow organ for the reception of fluid. *Urinary B.* receives the urine from the kidneys. *See* Gall bladder.

Blalock's operation. The subclavian artery is anastomosed to the pulmonary artery. Performed in cases of congenital pulmonary stenosis.

Blindness. Lack of sight. *Colour B.*, an inability to distinguish certain colours. *Cortical B.*, blindness due to a lesion of the visual centre in the brain. *Night B.*, or nyctalopia, vision subnormal at night, thought to be due to a deficiency of vitamin A in the diet. Snow *B.*, dimness of vission with pian and lacrimation due to the glare of sunlight upon snow. Word *B* ., in ability to recognize familiar written words owing to a lesion of the brain.

Blind spot. Point where the optic nerve enters the retina.

Blister. A collection of serum between the layers of the skin. A bleb, a vescle.

Blood. The red fluid which circulates through the heart, arteries, capillaries and veins, Blood consists of a pale yellowish albuminous fluid, called plasma, in which are carried numerous minute cells. There are the red blood cells, or crythrocytes, which hold the haemoglobin, carry oxygen and give to blood its red colour; and the white blood cells or leucocytes. The leucocytes are of various kinds, named as follows: polymorphonuclears or granulocytes, of three kinds, neutrophils, eosinophils, basophils; lymphocytes, small and large, and monocytes. In blood diseases abnormal forms appear and the total number and the ratio to each other of these various kinds differ. The blood also contains minute discs called platelets.

The functions of the blood are to carry to the tissues the water and nourishment which they require, to take off the waste products of their growth and activities, and to distribute heat equably through the body. In addition, the blood carries the antitoxins and other substances which defend the system against bacterial invasion, and certain other substances which are necessary for the general functions of the body or the individual functions of the various organs.

When blood is shed fibrinogen, a soluble protein in the plasma, is converted to an insoluble thread-like form, fibrin, which consititutes the clot. The change is affected by an enzyme, thrombin, which is not active in circulating blood, in which it exists as prothrombin. Prothrombin is converted to thrombin at the time of shedding blood by the action of a second enzyme, thrombokinase which is set free by the breaking-up of platelets. The process also requires the presence of calcium ions for its completion.

The figures igven below represent the approximate range of values for the constituents of the peripheral blood.

Red Cells

	SIIints	*Traditional Units*
Haemoglobin	12.0 to 18.0 g/dl	12 to 16 g per 100 ml
Red cells	3.9 to 6.5 × 10²/1	45. to 6.0 million per cu mm or mm²
Reticulocytes (newly formed red cells)	same	less than 1 per cent of total red cells
Mean cell volume (MCV)	same	75 to 95 cuμ is the average volume of a single red cell
Packed cell volume (PCV or haematocrit)	same	35 to 55 per cent
Mean cell diameter (MCD)	same	7.2μ
Mean cell haemoglobin (MCH)	same	20 to 32μg

White Cells

	S.I. Units	*Traditional Units*
Total white cells	5.0 to 10.0 × 10⁹/1	5,000 to 10,000 per cu mm or mm³

Neutrophils	same	60 to 70 per cent
Lymphocytes	same	25 to 35 per cent
Basophils	same	1 per cent
Eosionophils	same	1 to 4 per cent
Platelets (thrombocytes)	2.5 to 3.5×10^{11}/l	250,000 to 350.000 per cu mm or mm^3

Blood Chemistry

	S.I. Units	Traditional Units
pH	same	7.35 to 7.45
Urea	2 to 3 mmol/2	20 to 40 mg per 100 ml
Uric acid	0.10 to 0.40 mmol/l	1.5 to 6.5 mg per cent
Cholesterol	3.9 to 7.8 mmol/l	1.5 to 6.5 mg per cent
Bilirubin	3 to 20 µmoi/ï	0.2 to 1.2 mg per cent
Calcium	2.3 to 2.6 mmol/l	9.0 to 10.2 mg per cent
Phosphate	0.8 to 1.46 mmol/	2.5 to 4.5 mg per cent

Bicarbonate	20 to 28 mmol/l	20 to 28 mEq/litre
Fasting blood glucose	2.3 to 5.0 mmol/l	45 to 90 mg per cent
Potassium	3.5 to 5.5 mmol/l	3.3 to 5.5 mEq/litre
Sodium	135 to 145 mmol/l	135 to 145 mEq/litre
Total plasma Proteins	60 to 80g/l	6.0 to 8.0 g per cent
Albumin	35 to 55g/l	3.5 to 5.5g per cent
Globulin	15 to 30g/l	1.5 to 3.0 g per cent
Fibrinogen	2 to 4g/l	0.2 to 0.4 g per cent

Blood-brain barrier. Hypothetical barrier separating the blood from the parenchyma of the central nervous system.

Blood caste. Small shreds of coagulated blood found in the urine in certain cases of disease or injury of the kidney.

Blood count. Examination and enumeration microscopically of the various cells in the blood. A normal blood count would be, in an average healthy man between 20 and 40 years: *Red cells* - 4,000,000 to 5,000,000 per cubic milimetre; *White cells* 7,000 to 10,000. If the different forms of white cells are estimated, it is called a *differential white blood count* and the percentages are as fol-

lows: *polymorphonuclears* - 60 to 70 per cent;
eosinophils - 2 to 3 per cent; *large and small lymphocytes* - 20 to 25 per cent; *other rarer forms* - 4 to
8 per cent. *See* HAEMOGLOBIN, COLOUR INDEX,
EOSINOPHILIA, LEUCOCYTOSIS.

Blood grouping. For a blood transfusion it is essential that
the blood of the donor be compatible with that of the
patient. Blood grouping is decided according to the
presence or absence of certain agglutinogens in the cells,
two in number, A and B. The international nomenclature
of the different groups is as follows: AB, A, B, O.
Group AB are those who may receive blood from any
other group, and are called universal recipients. Group A
may recieve blood from Groups A and O. Group B may
receive blood from Groups B and O. Group O may
receive only from Group O. From the above it will be
seen that Group O can give blood to all other groups,
and therefore is a universal donor. Before transfusion a
direct match is always made between the red cells of the
donor and the serum of the recipient. Any clumping
together or agglutination of the cells which can be seen
even with the naked eye means incompatibility. The
Rhesus (Rh.) Factor. It has been recently shown that 85
per cent of human beings of most races posses this agglutinogen in their red cells, and so are termed 'Rh
positive'. The remaining 15 per cent, 'Rh negative', are
liable to form an anti-body (agglutinin) against the agglutinogen, if it is introduced into their circulation. It
may occur in an 'Rh negative' woman if she becomes
pregnant with a fetus whose blood cells are 'Rh positive'
or if an 'Rh negative' person is transfused with 'Rh posi-

tive blood.

Blood-letting. Bleeding, phlebotomy, venesection. The withdrawal of blood for therapeutic purposes from a vein.

Blood plasma. The fluid part of blood in which the cells are suspended.

Blood pressure. The pressure exerted by the blood in the vessels in which it is contained. It is taken in the brachial artery and estimated in terms of the number of milimetres pressure of mercury required, on the upper arm, just ot obliterate the pulse at the wrist. This figure is the *systolic b. pressure*. The average systolic pressure in a young adult is 100–120. The *diastolic b. pressure* is the pressure in the artery during the resting phase of the cardiac cycle, i.e. the lowest pressure. The average diastolic pressure is 70 to 90 in a young adult. It rises with age. High blood pressure is present in arteriosclerosis and some kinds of kidney and heart disease.

Blood sedimentation rate. 0.4 ml of a 3.8 per cent sol. of sodium citrate is drawn into a citringe. Blood is then taken into the syringe from a vein until the total quantity reaches 2ml mark. The blood and citrate are thoroughly mixed and then sucked into a standard pipette to make a column 200 mm high. The pipette is placed vertically and the column of fluid examined exactly one hour later. It is found that the red cells have sedimented leaving a clear supernatant fluid. In health the length of clear fluid on top varies from 1 to 5 mm. In active tuberculosis or other toxaemic states it may be 20 to 100 mm or more.

Blood serum. See SERUM.

Blood sugar. The amount of sugar normally in the blood is about 0.08 to 0.12 per cent or 80 to 120 mg per 100 ml of blood. This figure rises slightly after a meal, but not to more than about 180 mg. Above this figure, sugar leaks through into the urine. The blood sugar is raised in diabetes mellitus.

Blood transfusion. The transference of blood from a healthy individual to one suffering from a grave degree of anaemin due to either haemorrhage or disease. The donor must not have suffered from certain specified diseases and his blood must belong to the same or to a compatible group. *See* BLOOD GROUPUNG. Clotting is prevented by the addition of 3.8 per cent sodium citrate solution. The blood is taken from the median basilic or other suitable vein of the arm; the quantity is usually 500 ml. This is allowed to flow from the needle in the arm, along a piece of short tubing into a vacuum bottle containing citrate solution; all needles and tubing have previously been run through with citrate solution. The blood is injected into the patient by (1) the closed method, through a thick hollow needle or fine polythene tubing into the vein. (2) The vein of the patient is out down upon, isolated and lifted; an incision is made into it, a small cannula slipped into the opening and tied there. The blood is then slowly run in from a giving set through a drip cannula. After the cannula in the arm is withdrawn, the vein is tied above and below and the skin incision closed.

Blood urea. Normally about 30 mg per 100 ml of blood, or 0.03 per cent, rising to a higher figure with increasing age. An abnormal amount of urea present usually shows deficient kidney action.

Blood volume. The calculated amount of blood in the

whole body: About 5 litres in the normal adult.

Bloodless operation. An operation unaccopanied by loss of blood. In the case of operation on a limb the blood is expelled from the part operated upon by raising the limb and applying a tourniquet or by applying an elastic bandage.

Blue baby. A cyanosed infant, due to congenital cardiac defects called the tetralogy of Fallot.

Blue line on gums. This is seen near the margin in cases of lead poisoning and aids diagnosis. The line is interrupted where there are no teeth.

Blue stone, Copper sulphate.

BMR. Abbreviation for basal metabolic rate. *See* BASAL METABOLISM.

BNA. Abbreviation for *basle Nomina Anatomica*. Naming of anatomical terms agreed in Switzerland in 1895.

Bodecker index. The ratio between the number of tooth surfaces (five to a tooth) which are carious and the total number of surfaces of the teeth which could be affected.

Boeck's disease. *See* SARCOIDOSIS.

Böhler's iron. An iron heel incorporated in plaster of Paris when applied to the leg to permit walking.

Boil. Furuncle. A staphylococcal infection of the skin, causing inflammation round a hair follicle.

Bolus. A large round mass such as that of food before it is swallowed.

Bomb. An apparatus containing radium so that its rays may be applied to any desired part of the body.

Bone. Hard material forming the skeleton. It is made mainly of collagen impregnated with mineral substance, chiefly phosphate and calcium and contains bone cells or osteocytes. The hard outer part is compact tissue and the inner is cancellous tissue.

Bone graft. A portion of bone is transplanted to remedy a defect.

Bone marrow. Fatty substance contained within the marrow cavity of bones. In the flat bones, and with children in the long bones as well, the fat is replaced by active blood-forming tissue, which is responsible for production of the granular leucocytes, the red cells and platelets.

Boracic acid. Boric acid. A mild antiseptic used for irrigation of eyes, usual strength, half saturated solution.

Borax. Sodium biborate. A weak antiseptic. With glycerin and honey it is used as a soothing drug in inflammation of the mouth.

Borborygmus. Rumbling of intestinal flatus.

Boric acid. Boracic acid.

Bornholm disease. Epidemic diaphragmatic pleurodynia.

Boss. A projection.

Botallo's foramen. The foramen ovale in the atrial septum of the fetal heart.

Botulism. Food poisoning by Bacillus botulinus. Usually fatal.

Bougie. A slender solid instrument which is flexible and yielding, used for dilating contracted passages.

Bouillon. (1) A Broth or soup. (2) A liquid nutritive medium for culture purposes.

Bovine. Pertaining to or derived from the ox or cow.

Bowel. The intestine. The gut. It consists of the small and large intestine. The small intestine is about 20ft long and is divided into: (1) *Duodenum*, 12 in long; (2) *Jejunum*, about 8ft long; (3) *Ileum*, about 12ft long. The large intestine is about 5ft long and consists of (1) the *Caecum* with the *Vermiform Appendix*; (2) *Ascending Colon*, running up the right side; (3) *Transverse Colon*, running from right to left; (4) *Descending Colon*, running down left side; (5) *Sigmoid or Pelvic Colon*, passing to (6) *Rectum* which opens externally via (7) the *Anal Canal.*

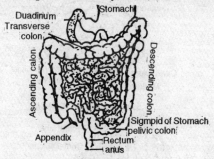

The bowel

Bow-leg. Genu varum.

Bowman's capsules. *See* MALPIGHIAN CORPUSCLES.

Boyle's law. At any given temperature, the volume of a given mass of gas varies inversely to the pressure it bears.

Bozeman's catheter. An intrauterine catheter grooved for ensuring the unobstructed return of fluid.

B.P. British Pharmacopoeia. *See* FORMULARY.

B.P.C. British Pharmaceutical Codex.

Brachial. Pertaining to the arm. *B. artery*, the main artery of the arm; it is a continuation of the axillary artery. *B neuralgia. Syn. B.* neuritis. Pain in arm due to pressure on the brachial plexus. B plexus, The plexus of nerves supplying the arm, forearm, and hand.

Brachium. The arm.

Bradycardia. Abnormally slow pulse. Occurs in heart block and head injuries.

Brain. The main integrating mass of nervous tissue situated in the skull. It may be divided into cerebral hemispheres, cerebellum and brain stem.

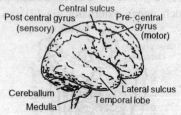

Central sulcus
Post central gyrus (sensory)
Pre- central gyrus (motor)
Cereballum
Medulla
Lateral sulcus
Temporal lobe

Lateral view of the brain

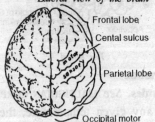

Frontal lobe
Cental sulcus
Parietal lobe
Occipital motor

11 the brain from above

Branchial. Pertaining to the gills. Thus *branchial cysts* are sometimes found in certain regions of the neck as vestiges of the gill stage of fetal development.

Braun's splint. A combined splint and extension apparatus for the lower limb.

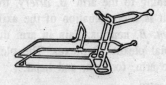

A Braun's splint

Breast. (1) The milksecreting gland. (2) The anterior surface of the thorax. *See* MAMMAE.

Breath. Air taken into and expelled from the lungs. *B. holding.* A behaviour disorder of infants and children. *B sounds*, the sounds heard by auscultation of the chest during respiration.

Breech. The buttocks. *B. persentation*, presentation of buttocks of fetus.

Bregma. *See* FONTANELLE.

Bright's disease. Disease of the kidney, characterized by proteinuria, casts, and oedema. Nephritis.

Brilliant green. Antiseptic dye used as a lotion, 1 in 1000, and as ointment 2 per cent.

Broad ligaments. The folds of peritoneum with the contained lymphatics, blood vessels, Fallopin tubes, etc., which pass outwards on each side of the uterus.

Broadbent's sign. Retraction of the lower left part of the chest wall when the pericardium is adherent.

Broca's area. The motor speech area normally on the left side of the brain in right-handed people.

Brodie's abscess. Chronic abscess of bone. The tibia is most commonly affected.

Bromidrosis. Offensive sweating, most common in the feet.

Bromism. Poisoning by bromides. Symptoms: red, papular rash, conjunctivitis.

Bronchi. The two tubes into which the trachea divides, opposite the upper border of the fifth dorsal vertebra.

Bronchial tubes. The smaller tubes into which the bronchi divide in the lung.

Bronchiectasis. A disease of the bronchial tubes in which they become dilated and usually secret offensive pus in large quantities. Treatment, postural drainage, antibiotics lobectomy, pneumonectomy.

Bronchiole. A minute bronchial tube.

Bronchiolitis, Inflammation of the bronchil

Bronchitis. Inflammation of the brochioles tubes.

Bronchocele. A diverticulum of a bronchus.

Bronchogenic. Originating from a bronchus.

Bronchography. Instillation of radioopaque dye in the bronchi, so that they are apparent on x-ray.

Broncholith. A bronchial calculus.

Bronchomycosis. Infection of the bronchi by fungus infection of lungs.

Bronchophony. Resonance of patient's voice as heard on auscultating the bronchi.

Broncho-pleural fistula. An opening between a bronchus and the pleural cavity found in disease.

Broncho-pneumonia, Pneumonia, beginning in the bronchioles, affecting scattered lobules of the lung and also the finest or capillary bronchioles.

Bronchoscope. An instrument for seeing into the main bronchi.

Bronchoscopy. Examination of the bronchi with a bronchoscope.

Bronchospirometry. The measurement of the capacity of a lung or one of its lobes.

Brow. The forehead. *B. presentation.* An unfavourable but unusual presentation in labour at the uterine orifice. The mento-vertical diameter, which is 13.0cm, presents.

Brownian movement. Oscillatory movement seen under the microscope in fine particles suspended in a liquid.

Brucella abortus bovinus. The bacterium from an infected cow causing undulant fever.

Brucella melitensis. Bacterium from an infected goat whose milk causes Malta fever in man.

Brucellosis. Infection with an organism of the Brucella group.

Bruise. A contusion. The skin is not broken but is discoloured due to bleeding in the underlying tissues.

Bruit. The French for 'sound', used with regard to sounds heard in auscultation.

Brunhilde virus. A strain of poliomyelitis virus.

Brunner's glands. Glands of the duodenum.

Bubo. Inflammatory swelling of glands, particularly of groin.

Bubonic plague. Oriental plague, which in some forms is characterized by the development of buboes.

Buccal, Pertaining to the mouth.

Buccinator. The muscle of the cheek; one of the muscles of mastication.

Buerger's disease. Thromboanfitis obliterans. Rare disease of blood vessels resulting in reduction of blood supply to extremities.

Buffer. A substance allowing only slight changes of pH when an acid or alkali is added to it, *e.g.* sodium bicarbonate in blood and tissue fluids.

Bulb. A rounded expansion of an organ.

Bulbar palsy. Paralysis due to disease of medulla oblongata.

Bulimia. Morbid hunger.

Bullae. Large blisters.

Buller's shield. Used to protect the sound eye from discharge poured from the infected one in contagious ophthalmia. It consists of sticking plaster and a watch glass.

Bundle of His. *See* ATRIOVENTRICULAR BUNDLE.

Bunion. Inflammation of a bursa situated over the metatarsophalangeal joint of the great toe.

Burette. A graduated tube for measuring a reagent.

Burns. Burns are of different degrees according to the depth of tissue involved. Those of the first degree show redness, of the second degree, blistering; third-degree burns involve the entire thickness of the skin fourth-degree burns show charring of muscle and bone. The first-aid treatment is to exclude air by applying a dressing soaked in a solution of soda bicarb. or saline, and to treat the shock.

Burr hole. Circular hole out in the cranium to allow access to the brain.

Bursa. A small sac interposed between movable parts. *B mucosa.* A sac lined with synovial membrane secreting synovial fluid.

Bursitis. Inflammation of a bursa.

Buttock. Breech. Nates.

Byssinosis. A type of pneumoconiosis caused by inhalation of cotton dust.

Caecostomy. Operation to provide an opening into the caecum through the abdominal wall.

Caecum. The blind intestine, a cul-de-sac at the commencement of the large intestine.

Caesarean section. Delivery of the fetus through an incision in the abdominal and uterine walls.

Caisson disease Also known as 'the bends'. The effect on those working under a heavier atmospheric pressure than normal, *e.g.* in deep mines or under water. Return to normal pressure should be effected gradually or nitrogren bubbles form in the blood and tissues.

Calamine. Zinc carbonate used as an astringent.

Callus. A new bony deposit around a fracture. Some of this is absorbed, the remainder develops into new bone which repairs the fracture.

Canal of Nuck. A narrow passage along which the round ligament passes to the region of the pubes, it is sometimes the seat of inguinal hernia and occasionally of cysts.

Canaliculus. A small canal or groove, e.g. (1) the hairlike passage leading from the edge of the eyelid to the lacrimal sac. (2) One of the minute spaces in a cancellou bone.

Cancer. A general term used to describe various types of malignant disease.

Cannabis indica. Indian hemp, hashish; a soporific and cerebral stimulant. One of the drugs controlled by the Misuse of Drugs Act.

Cannula. Surgical name for a metal tube used to withdraw fluid from a cavity.

Capilaries. The network of microscopic vessels which communicated with the arterioles and the venules. The walls are formed of a single layer of endothelium.

Capillarity. Effect of surface tension causing liquid to rise up inside a small tube.

Carbolic acid. Phenol. A powerful antiseptic obtained from coal tar. Highly poisonous. Used in a solution of 2.5% to 5% as a disinfectant.

Carbon monoxide poisoning. Poisoning by inhalation of carbon monoxide, *e.g.* from coal gas or motor vehicle exhaust. Symptoms begin as giddiness and singing of ears, then lividity of face and body; later, owing to combination of the gas with the blood, the patient may have a rosy tinge; loss of muscular power; violent action of heart and lungs; fixed dilated pupils convulions, coma or asphyxia. *Treatment:* fresh air, oxygen and artificial respiration if necessary.

Carboxyhaemoglobin. A compound of carbon monoxide and haemoglobin formed in coal-gas poisoning.

Carbuncle. Severe staphylococcal inflammation of an area of skin and subcutaneous tissue. There is necrosis and liquefaction of the cubcutaneous tissue and several points of discharge.

Carcinogenic. Term applied to substances producing or

ɪ redisposing to cancer.

Carcinoma. A type of cancer growing from epithelial tissue. One mode of spread is by way of the lymph channels, and therefore glands near, and at a distance, are involved.

Carcinomatosi. Disseminated malignant disease.

Cardi. (1) The heart. (2) The aperture between the oesophagus and the stomach.

Cardiac. Relating to the heart. *C. catheterization.* Investigation to diagnose certain heart conditions. A catheter is introduced through a vein in the arm into the chambers of the heart from which pressure recordings can be obtained. *C. massage.* Squeezing the heart rhythmically to simulate the normal heart beat in an attempt to restart the circulation, having first gained access to the heart through an incision in the chest. *External. C. massage.* Pressure on the chest with patient lying flat on back. The heart is rhythmically pressed netween the front and back of the thoracic cage.

Cardiac cycl. The changes in the heart to produce one heart beat.

Cardiogram. The tracing obtained by the use of the cardiograph.

Cardiograph. An instrument which records the movements of the heart.

Cardiology, The study of the heart and circulatory disorders.

Cardiomyotomy. Operation to relieve muscular spasm at the lower end of the oesophagus.

Castle's factors. Two factors, one in gastric juice, the other in certain foods, providing the anti-anaemic factor.

CAT. Computerized axial tomography. The technique of examining body section in the axial plane using very sophisticated equipment.

Catalepsy. A period of trance, during which the limbs remain in any position in which they are placed.

Catharsis. Emotional relief brought about by the conscious realization of suppressed desires.

Cathartic. A drastic purge.

Catheter. Instrument used for the passage of fluids; usually from the bladder where there is urethral obstruction, *Nasal c.* (Ryle's tube). Used for the administration of fluid feeds. The tube passes through the nose down the throat into the stomach. *Eustachian c.* A special tube used to inflate the pharyngo-tympanic tube (Eustachian tube).

Cauda equina. The bundle of sacral and lumbar nerves at the base of the spinal cord.

Caudal analgesia. Regional anaesthesia of the rectum and perineum produced by injecting local anaesthetics into the sacral canal through at birth.

Caul. Fetal membranes about the face and head of some infants at birth.

Cauliflower growth. Term applied to the shape of a tumour growing from a surface.

Causalgia. Pain referred to in the distribution of a cutaneous nerve which persists long after an injury to that nerve. Often follows herpes zoster (shingles). The cause is not known.

Cautery. Application of heated metal to living tissue in oder to destroy it or to arrest haemorrhage. Diathermy is used during operations to arrest bleeding and to destroy tissue when excising malignant growths.

Cavernous respiration. A hollow sound, heard on auscultation, when there is a cavity in the lung.

Cavernous sinus. A blood sinus on the body of the sphenoid bone.

Cavitation. Process whereby cavities are formed.

Cavity of pelvis. The space between the pelvic inlet and outlet.

Central nervous system. Abbreviation CNS. Generally term incorporating the brain and spinal cord, as opposed to the peripheral nervous system, which includes the nerves and sensory receptors outside the brain and spinal cord.

Centriole. Small granule situated just outside the nuclear membrane and found in many resting cells. Just before mitosis this granule divides and at mitosis the two resulting centrioles move apart and form the poles of the spindle.

Centromere. A structure formed during nuclear division; a spindle- attachment. The region of the chromosome which attaches it to the spindle which is composed of long protein molecules passing between chromosomes and the centriole when the cell is dividing.

Centrosome. Region of differentiated cytoplasm in which the centriole is situated.

Cephalhaematoma. A subperiosteal haemorrhage on head of an infant, usually due to pressure during a long labour. It is gradually absorbed.

Cephalic version. The production artificially of a cephalic prsentation, from, a breech presentation or transverse lie.

Cephalometry. Estimation of the size of the head of a fetus, usually by radiographic means.

Cerebellum. Outgrowth from the hind-brain overlying the medulla oblongata. Concerned with the co-ordination of movement.

Cerebral haemorrhage. Rupture of an artery of the brain, due to either high blood pressure or disease of artery. Escape of brain tissue, and paralysis occurs of that side of the body which is opposite to the injured side of the brain. If the haemorrhage has occurred on the left side of the brain, the speech is affected.

Cerebral palsy. A condition in which the control of the motor system is affected due to a lesion in the brain resulting from a birth injury or pre-natal defect. The popular term is 'spastic'.

Cerebral thrombosis. Thrombus formation in vessels supplying the brain generally resulting in cerebrovascular accident.

Cerebration. Activity of the brain. Thinking.

Cerebrospinal fever. Epidemic meningitis of the brain and spinal cord, caused by the meningococcus. The fever is often accompanied by a rash; hence the popular name 'spotted fever'.

Cerebrospinal fluid. The clear watery fluid which lies in the subarachnoid space, surrounding the brain and spinal cord. It also fills the cavities or ventricles of the brain. Its function is to protect the brain and spinal cord.

Cerebrovascular accident. General term referring to cerebral embolism thrombosis or haemorrhage.

Cerebrum. The larger part of the brain occupying the cranium.

Cerumen. Waxy secretion of the external auditory meatus.

Cervical. Pertaining to the neck or cervix of the uterus *C rib*. Outgrowth from the seventh cervical vertebra, passing out and down to join rib below. It may press on nerve trunks of the arm giving rise to tingling and pins and needles in hand and fingers. *C. spondylosis.*

Degenerative changes in the interverbral discs of he cervical spine with associated secondary osteo-arthritic changes in the intervertebral joints of the neck.

Cervicectomy. Excision of the cervix uteri.

Cervicitis. Inflammation of the cervix of the uterus.

Cervix. A neck. *C. uteri.* the neck of the uterus. The lowest third of the uterus, about one inch in length. It is traversed by a canal which opens into the vagina.

Cestoda. Tapeworms.

Cetavlon. Official name Cetrimide, B.P., abbreviation CTAB, a detergent with antiseptic action, used as a 1% solution.

Cetrimion. Quaternary ammonium compound used to cleanse skin, etc.

Chalazion. Meibomian cyst. A small retention cyst in the eyelid, due to blocking of a meibomian follicle.

Chancre. Syphilitic ulcer of the first stage; occurs at the site of infection. Contagious.

Chemotherapy. Healing by chemical means, administration of drugs. A term which was commonly applied to the use of sulphonamide drugs. Nowadays used to define treatment of malignant disease by cytotoxic drugs.

Cholangiogram. X-ray showing the biliary system.

Cholangitis. Inflammation of the biliary system.

Cholecystectomy. Removal of the gall bladder.

Cholecystenterostomy. Operation for forming an artificial communication between the gall bladder and the intestine.

Cholecystitis. Inflammation of the gall bladder.

Cholecystogastrostomy. An operation for forming an artificial communication between the gall bladder and the stomach.

Cholecystography. X-ray examination of the gall bladder, after it has been rendered opaque to x-rays by drugs such as pheniodol. Low fat meal 15 hours before, then no futher food allowed but water as desired. The first skiagram taken is twelve hours later, and two further ones at intervals of $2\frac{1}{2}$ to 3 hours. Some times a meal rich in fat is ordered before taking the later pictures, in order that the emptying power of the gall bladder may be observed.

Cholecystolithiasis. A stone or stones in the gall bladder.

Cholecystostom. Operation for making the gall bladder open to the exterior.

Chromosomes. When a cell divides, the genetic material present in the nucleus becomes segregated into thread-shaped bodies which are visible under the microscope. These are known as chromosomes and consist of connected strands of DNA molecules known as genes. In man there are 46 chromosomes per cell: 22 pairs of *sex chromosomes*; females have two X chromosomes, males one X and one Y. The Y chromosome is shorter than the X chromosome.

Chronic. A disease from which complete cure is never obtained and which tends to worsen.

Chvostek's sign. A spasm of the facial muscles produced by tapping the facial nerve. This sign is present in tetany.

Circle of Willis. Circular intercommunication of arteries supplying the brain.

Ciculation. Arterial blood received into the left atrium passes through the mitral valve to the left ventricle. It then passes into the aorta and through its smaller branches to the capillaries—into smaller veins, then larger, until on reaching the superior and inferior venae cavae it passes into the right atrium. *Pulmonary circulation*. The venous blood which is received into right atrium passes through the tricuspid valve into the right ventricle. From there into the pulmonary artery, which divides into two branches, one going to each lung. The artery divides in the lung into capillaries, and here, by means of the haemoglobin in the red cells, takes up oxygen from the inspired air. Oxygenated blood returns to the heart by the four pulmonary veins, two from each lung entering the left atrium. *Portal circulation*. Veins from the pancreas, spleen, stomach, intestines, unite behind the pancreas and form the prortal tube or vein. This takes blood, rich in the products of digestion, to the liver where into divides it smaller vessels and capillaries. Blood leaves the liver by the hepatic veins which enter the inferior vena cava.

Circumcision. Surgical removal of the foreskin.

Circumduction. Circular movement of a limb.

Circumflex nerve. This arises from the brachial plexus to supply the deltoid and teres minor muscles.

Cisternal puncture. A puncture made with a hollow needle at the nape of the neck into a space called the cisterna magna which contains cerebrospinal fluid. Used when the fluid cannot be obtained by lumbar puncture.

Clubbing. The appearance of fingers and sometimes toes when the normal angle at the base of the nail is lost. It results from hyperplasia of connective tissue. Clubbing is associated with longstanding respiratory or cardiovascular disease.

Coagulase test. Test used of identification of pathogenic staphylococci which depend on the demonstration of the enzyme coagulase which breaks down fibrinogen and clots plasma.

Coagulation, Thickening of a fluid into curds or clots. Almost always applied to blood.

Cocaine. A powerful local anaesthetic, much used in ophthalmology. It enlarges the pupil of the eye. Included in the Misuse of Drugs Act.

Cocainism. Chronic poisoning from indulgence in the drug.

Coccus. Any spheroidal-shaped micro-organism. *See* BACTERIA.

Coccydynia. Pain in the coccyx.

Coccyx. The tail-like termination of the spine.

Cohlea. The spiral cavity of the internal ear, containing the nerve endings of the eighth cranial or auditory nerve.

Cock-up splints. For hand and wrist. Usually made of metal.

A cock-up spling

Cod-liver oil. *Oleum Morrhuae*; contains vitamin D. Used in the prevention and treatment of rickets.

Coeliac. Related to the abdominal cavity.

Coeliac diseases. A condition commencing in early childhood, associated with deficient absorption of fat from the intestines, resulting in the passage of loose, bulky pale, offensive stools, abdominal enlargement, wasting and retarded development.

Coelioscopy. Also known as peritoneoscopy. Examination of the abdominal contents as follows: a small incision is made through the abdominal wall under a local anaesthetic. Air is passed into the peritoneal cavity and the contents viewed by means of a laparoscope. This method may be used when an exploratory laparotomy is unjustifiable.

Coffee ground vomit. Vomit which contains partly digested blood.

Cognition. Awareness. Part of a mental process. There is cognition when there is perception or memory of a material thing or idea.

Coitus, Sexual intercourse.

Colchicum. Drug used in the treatment of gout.

Colectomy. The operation of removing the colon.

Colic, Severe abdominal pain due to muscular spasm of a hollow viscus frequently caused by obstruction. *Biliary colic.* Intense pain due to lodging of a gallstone in the cystic or common bile duct. Sudden relief when it passes into duodenum. *Intestinal colic.* Severe pain in the abdomen due to irritation of the gut as in food poisoning. *Renal colic.* Same when due to a stone in the pelvis of kidney blocking up upper end of ureter. Uterine colic. Spasmodic contractions of the uterus as it endeavours to expel its contents.

Collapse. Severe sudden prostration symptoms: see SHOCK. *Massive c.,* of one or more lobes of the lung, may result from a chest wound. *C. of the lungs.* Lack of air in previously expanded ait tissue.

Colles' fracture. Transverse fracture of the radius just above the wrist with displacement of the hand backwards and outwards.

Colles' law. A woman may breast-feed her baby and this child being syphilitic may affect others and yet apparently not the mother. The explanation is —the mother is already affected, not yet showing any signs of the disease, but her Wassermann will be positive, and later in life she will show some signs of late tertiary syphilis, *e.g.* gummata, GPI or tabes.

Collodion. Pyroxylin dissolved in alcohol and ether; used in surgery to form a false skin for clean wounds. Highly inflammable.

Colostrum. A milky fluid flowing from the breasts the first two or three days after confinement, before the true milk comes.

Colotomy, An incision into the colon.

Colour blindness. Inability to distinguish certain colours, knows sometimes as Daltonism.

Colour index, Is a measure of the amount of haemoglobin contained in each red cell, compared to the normal amount. It is calculated thus:

$$\frac{\text{Haemoglobin percentage}}{\text{Red cell percentage}} \quad \text{Normal} \quad \frac{100}{100} = 1$$

Colpitis. Inflammation of the vagina.

Colpocele. A tumour or hernia in the vagina.

Colpohysterectomy. Removal of the uterus through the vagiva.

Colpoperineorrhaphy. Operation for repairing a torn vagina and perineum.

Confluent smallpox. A severe form of smallpox in which the individual papules coalesce.

Constipation. Infrequent bowel action, leading to the rectum being filled with hard faeces.

Constitutional. Affecting the whole body, not local.

Contraceptives, oral. Drugs, usually combined oestrogens and progestogens, which inhibit ovulation. They prevent blastocyst implantation and make cervical mucus unfavourable to sperm migration.

Contracted pelvis. A pelvis is contracted if any of its diameters is shorter than normal (*See* CONJUGATE and DIAMETERS). The commonest form of contraction is the *simple flat* pelvis in which the true conjugate is the only diameter materially shortened. Other common forms are the *generally contracted* or *small round* pelvis: and the *generally contracted* or small round pelvis. The obliquely distorted, the triradiate, the osteomalacic, the spondylolisthetic and others are rare. A contracted pelvis may lead to difficulty during delivery.

Contre-coup. Injury through transmission of force of the blow, remote form original point of contact.

Coombs' test. Coombs' reagent detects the presence of any antibody coating the red cell, i.e. in a newborn baby with haemolytic disease and following a mis-matched blood transfusion.

Coronary. Encircling as a vessel. *C. arteries* supply the heart muscle; narrowing and spasm of these produce angina pectoris. There are also coronary arteries in the stomach. *C. sinus,* a passage for the venous blood into the right atrium.

Corpus luteum. A temporary organ secreting the hormone progesterone which favours the establishment and continuity of a pregnancy. It is formed under the influence of luteinizing hormone of the pituitary, by growth of the wall of Graafian follicle after ovulation. If ovulation does not result in fertilization the corpus luteum degenerates, but if fertilization occurs, the corpus luteum persists.

Corrigan's pulse. Known also as water-hammer pulse, occurs in aortic regurgitation. The artery distends forcibly and then appears to empty suddenly and completely.

Corrosive sublimate. Perchloride of mercury. powerful, very poisionous antiseptic. For douches is used in strengths of 1 in 1,000 to 1 in 10,000. Itself colourless, it is generally coloured blue to distinguish it.

Coupling. Abnormal heart beat which occurs in overdose of digitalis. The normal heart beat is followed by an extra ventricular contraction (ventricular extra-systole). The latter may be too weak to transmit a pulse.

Cowper's glands. Two small glands near the bulb of the urethra in male.

Coxsackie virus. Group of viruses which may cause epidemic myalgia (Bornholm disease) and benign lymphocytic meningitis, and possibly other relatively mild diseases.

Cresol. An antiseptic, similar to phenol, and obtained from coal-tar.

Cretinism. Congenital deficient thyroid secretion, causing impaired mentality, small, stature, coarseness of skin and hair and deposition of fat on the body. Treated early with thyroid extract, great improvement may result.

Crohn's disease. Chronic form of enteritis affecting the terminal part of the ileum, Syn. regional ileitis.

Croup. Dyspnoea and stridor due to obstruction of the larynx. It may be due to inflammation, or spasm of the muscles.

Crush syndrome. As the result of extensive crushing of muscles, toxic substances pass into the circulation which cause the medullary circulation of the kidney to be opened up so that blood is diverted from the glomeruli in the renal cortex. This results in oliguria.

Crutch paralysis. Caused by pressure on the axillary nerves and vessels by a crutch.

Curare. A poison derived from a South American plant. It paralyses motor nerves. Used by anaesthetists to produce muscular relaxation, thus reducing the amount of anaesthetic required.

Cushing's disease. Adenoma of pituitary with hypersecretion of ACTH resulting in adrenal cortical overactivity.

Cushing's syndrome. Syndrome due to oversecretion of adrenocortical hormones and characterized by moonface, redistribution of body fat, polycythaemia, hirsutism, acne, amenorrhoea, osteoporosis, glycosuria, hypertension, purpura, muscular weakness and occasionally mental derangement.

Cyanosis. Blue appearance; due to deficient oxygenation of the blood. It occurs in heart failure, diseases of the respiratory tract, and congenital heart disease.

Cyclotomy. Incision through the ciliary body of the eye.

Cystectomy. Removal of the urinary bladder.

Cystic disease of the lung. Congenital disease in which the pancreas is first affected and then the lung.

Cystic duct. The duct leading from the gall bladder to the common bile duct.

Cysticercosis. Normally the cysticercus stage of the tapeworm occurs in the pig. Occasionally it develops in the muscle or nervous system of man producing serious symptoms, *e.g.* epilepsy.

Cystine. A sulphur-containing amino-acid.

Cystitis. Inflammation of the urinary bladder.

Cystitome. Knife used by ophthalmic surgeion in operation for cataract.

Cystobubonocele. Hernia involving the bladder.

Cystoscope. An instrument for examining the bladder.

Cystostomy. Operation of producing an opening from the bladder to the exterior.

Cystotomy. Incision of the bladder or division of the anterior capsule of the lens of the eye.

Cytamen. cyanocobalamin.

Cytology. The study of cells. *Exfoliative c.* The study of shed cells used in the diagnosis of pre-malignant disease.

Cytometer. An instrument for counting cells, usually of the blood.

Cytoplasm. Protoplasm.

Cytotoxic. Substance which damages cells. *C. drugs.* Used in malignant disease to destroy cancer cells.

Dacryadenitis. Inflammation of the lacrimal gland.

Dacryocystitis. Inflammation of the tear sac.

Dacryocystorhinostomy. Operation to establish a communication between the tear (lacrimal) sac and the nose.

Dacryolith. Stone in the lacrimal duct.

Dacryoma. Benign tumour arising from lacrimal epithelium.

Dactyl. A digit of the hand or foot.

Dactylion. Webbed fingers or toes.

Dactylitias. Inflammation of the fingers or toes. Generally used of the bones only.

Dactylology. Talking by the fingers; deaf and dumb language.

Dakin's solution. An antiseptic solution containing sodium hypochlorite and boric acid used to irrigate wounds.

Daltonism. Colour blindness.

Dandruff. A scaly condition of the scalp.

DDT. A synthetic insecticide.

Deaf mute. An individual who is both deaf and dumb.

Deafness. Lack of hearing.

Deamination. The breaking down of aminoacids in the liver.

Debility. Weakness, loss of power.

Debridement. Thorough cleansing of a wound and excision of the edges.

Decalcification. Loss or removal of calcium salts from bone.

Decapitation. The operation of severing the fetal head from the body, very occasionally necessary in cases of obstructed labour.

Decapsulation. Removal of the capsule of an organ, *e.g.* of the kidney.

Decidua. The thickned lining of the uterus formed to receive the fertilized ovum. As the ovum grows larger, the decidua covering it is called the *decidua reflexa;* the part where it is attached to the uterine wall and which later becomes the placenta, the *decidua basalis;* while that lining the rest of the uterine cavity is the *decidua* vera.

Decompensation. Failure of compensation, as of the heart.

Decompression. An operation performed to relieve internal pressure, *e.g.* trephining of the skull. *D. sickness.* Caisson disease.

Decortication. Removal of the cortex or external covering from an organ, *e.g.* of the cerebrum or of the kidney. *D. pulmonary,* pleurectomy: removal of one or more ribs and the visceral layer of the pleura.

Decubitus. The recumbent or horizontal position.

Decussation. (1) An interlacing or crossing of fellow parts. (2) The point at which the crossing occurs. *D. of the pyramids.* The crossing of the motor fibres from one side of the medulla to the other.

Defaecation. Means the act of evacuating the bowels.

Defibrillator. Apparatus which applies electrical impulses to the heart. Designed to stop fibrillation and restore the normal cardiac cycle.

Deficiency diseases. Due to an inadequate supply of vitamins in the diet, *e.g.* rickets, scurvy, beriberi.

Degeneration. Deterioration in structure or function of tissue when the structural changes are marked, descriptive terms are sometimes used, *e.g.* colloid, fatty, hyaline, etc.

Deglutition. Refers to the act of swallowing.

Deltoid. The muscle which covers the prominence of the shoulder.

Delusion. A false idea, entirely without foundation in the facts of the environment.

Demarcation. The marking of a boundary. *Line of d.*, red lines which forms between dead and living tissue in gangrene.

Dementia. Feebleness of the mental faculties, inconsequent ideas. A form of insanity. An acquired condition. *D. praecox*, schizophrenia.

Dendron dendrite. A protoplasmic filament of nerve cell through which synaps occurs.

Dengue. A virus disease of the tropice, transmitted by mosquitoes and characterised by faver, headache, pains in the limbs, and a rash.

Denis Browne splints. A number of splints designed to correct congenital deformity, as that of the hip, bear this surgeon's name. His padded metal splints to correct congenital talipes equinovarus are widely used.

Dens. A tooth.

Dental. Pertaining to the teeth.

Dentine. The substance which forms the body of a tooth.

Dentition. Teething.

Denture. A set of artificial teeth.

Deodorant. deodórizer. Destroyer of smells; the chief deodorants are chloride of lime, sulphurous acid, nitrous acid, chlorophyll, iodoform, scents, and fumigating pastilles. They are all more or less disinfectants.

Deoxycorticosterone. A constituent of suprarenal cortex extract, prescribed in Addison's disease.

Depersonalization. A neurotic state when the person feels that he has no reality in existence but is only an onlooker at his own behaviour and actions.

Depilatory. An agent for removing superfluous hairs from the body.

Depression. A feeling of gloom due to dis-appointment, loss or failure. In *reactive depression*, due to stress, the patient does not lose touch with reality. *Endogenous depression* is a psychotic state and there is usually a predisposition to it in the person's make-up. He then loses all touch with reality and needs expert help. *Involutional depression* occasionally occurs at the menopau.

Dermatitis. Inflammation of the skin. The numerous causes may be of external or internal origin. Some common external irritants are dyes, metals, disinfectants, flowers.

Dermatology. The science of the skin and its diseases.

Dermatosis. Any skin disease.

Dialysis. The separation of certain substances form a mixture by passing the latter through a membrane. Usually applied to dialysis of blood to remove toxic waste in cases of renal insufficiency (kidney machine).

Diamorphine. An alkaloid obtained by the action of acetic anhydride on morphine. It allays cough, induces sleep and does not leave the depressing after-effects of morphia, but its narcotic action is less. (*syn.* Heroin) Addiction is a constant risk.

Diapedesis. The passage of leucocytes through the walls of blood- vessels. It occurs in inflammation.

Diaphragmatic hernia. Herniation of abdominal viscera through the diaphragm into the chest. Usually due to a congenital defect of the diaphragm. Hiatus hernia is an acquired form in adults.

Diaphysis. The middle part of long bones: the shaft, *cf.* epiphysis.

Diathermy. The passage of high frequency electric current through a tissue. Because of the electrical resistance of the tissue, heat is generated. This is diffuse when large electrodes are used, as in physiotherapy. Tissues may be cauterized by using a small electrode. Diathermy is used so that tissues are destroyed. *e.g.* as in removal of superficial new growths. It is also used as a cautery to arrest bleeding.

Diathesis. Constitutional disposition to a particular disease.

Dicrotic, pulse. Having two beats. Usually applies to secondary pulse wave due to the closure of semilunar valves since, when this is marked as in conditions associated with vasodilatation, *e.g.* high fever, it gives the impression of a double pulse.

Didactyle. Having only two fingers, or two toes.

Didymitis. Inflammation of the testicle.

Dielectric. The non-conducting material separating the conducting surface in an electrical condenser.

Diet. A pattern of food intake developed according to physiological need, availability and individual preference.

The human does not eat nutrients but food and the type of food eaten varies a great deal from culture to culture. However, certain basic nutrients are necessary for the production of energy, for adequate growth, the replacement of tissues and the maintenance of health.

The basic nutrients include:

1. Carbohydrates
2. Proteins
3. Fats
4. Vitamins
5. Minerals

The first three groups of these nutrients are energy-giving foods and the energy value of a diet is measured in kilojoules (SI unit). 4.186 kilojoules = 1 Calorie (kilocalorie). Energy requirements vary greatly according to sex, age and degree of activity.

Composition of some common foodstuffs per ounce (approx. 30 grams)

	Kilojoules	Protein grames	Fats grams	Carbohydrate grams
Bread	306	2.2	0.2	15.5
Potato	87	0.6	–	4.6
Sugar	452	–	–	26.6
Butter	883	0.1	23.4	–
Cheese	490	7.1	9.8	–
Egg	188	3.5	3.3	0.3
Milk	71	0.9	1.0	1.2
Bacon	536	3.1	12.8	–
Beef	373	4.2	8.0	–
Apple	50	0.1	–	3.0
Orange	42	0.2	–	2.2

APPENDIX 3

1. Carbohydrates

These contain carbon, hydrogen, and oxygen. Carbohydrates may be eaten as starch or as sugars. Sugars may be disaccharides or monosaccharides. The disaccharides are sucrose, containing one molecule of glucose and one of fructose; maltose, which contains two molecules of glucose; and lactose, which contains glucose and galactose. During digestion carbohydrates are broken down to the monosaccharides glucose, fructose and galactose. These are used in the body for the production of energy or stored as glycogen.

Carbohydrate is the only nutrient in sugar but is also present in such foods as bread, potatoes, rice and pasta. In these foods there are other nutrients including protein and vitamins.

The carbohydrates in the food supply from 50% to 80% of the total daily intake of energy. In wealthier countries fat and protein account for a relatively greater proportion but in poorer countries a larger proportion of energy is obtained from carbohydrates.

1 Gram carbohydrates gives 17 kJ

2. Proteins

These contain oxygen, hydrogen, nitrogen and sometimes, sulphur. They are necessary to the body for growth and repair. Opinions about the amount of protein necessary daily for a human differ widely and the amount suggested has varied from 40 grams to 100 grams. At present in the United Kingdom it is recommended that a fully grown adult should eat between 60 and 70 grams of protein a day which will supply about 10% of his total daily intake of colories. It is possible that humans would be healthier with a smaller amount of protein in the diet. Pregnant and lactating mothers need more protein than other adults.

Protein is made up of 23 amino-acids and of these 8 are called 'essential' amino-acids and a further two are 'essential' in children. The term 'essential' is used because the body is unable to synthesise these amino-acids and must have them in the food. Proteins were formerly known as first class or animal proteins which contained all the essential amino-acids and second class or vegetable proteins which contained some of the essential amino-acids. This categorisation has now stopped because it is realised that a varied intake of vegetable proteins including cereals and pulses can contain all the essential amino-acids. The quantity of vegetable protein that needs to be eaten is very much greater than animal protein and this can be a disadvantage.

Protein is used in the body for growth and repair and any excess is used up for energy or stored as fat.

1 gram protein gives 17 kJ

3. Fats

All fats are made up of a mixture of glycerol and fatty acids but the characteristics of the fatty acids differ. A fatty acid is formed from a chain of carbon atoms with hydrogen and oxygen. A saturated fatty acid is one in which all the bonds between the carbon atoms are single. A mono-saturated fatty acid is one in which one bond is double; a poly-unsaturated fatty acid is one in which there are two or more double bonds.

Fat is found in dairy products such as milk, cream, cheese and butter; but it is also present in and around meat, in nuts, pulses and in some fish including herring and salmon.

There are three poly-unsaturated fatty acids essential for

health and these are linoleic acid, linolenic acid and arachidonic acid.

The amount of fat that is necessary in the diet for health is not known. Cultural factors and the family income cause a wide variation in intake.

Fats are emulsified by the bile salts in the digestive tract and then broken down by lipase into glycerides, glycerol and fatty acids.

Fats form the main supply of stored energy in the body. When it is metabolised one gram of fat produces twice as many calories as a gram of protein or a gram of carbohydrate. Fat is also a source of vitamins A, D, E and K.

1 gram fat gives 38 kJ

4. Vitamins

These are a small but necessary part of the diet. The results of vitamin deficiencies were recognised in most cases before the chemical structure of the vitamin had been established. They were called A, B, C, etc. but this, in the light of later knowledge, has led to some confusion in the nomenclature.

Fat Slouble Vitamins

Vitamin A is supplied to the body in food as retinol and carotene. It is present in animal fats such as halibut and cod liver oil, milk, butter and cheese. It is also present in carrots and green vegetables with dark green leaves such as spinach.

2,500 International Units (IU) are necessary each day. Deficiency causes night blindness, hardening of the skin and the covering of the eye which can cause blindness. A deficiency is rare in the developed countries.

An excess of vitamin A, which can occur if children are given too large an amount, can cause irritability, loss of appetite, an itching skin and swellings over the bones.

Vitamin D is supplied to the body in animal fats including milk, butter and cheese. It can also be made by the body when the skin is exposed to ultraviolet light.

The recommended daily intake of vitamin D for infants is 400 International Units and for adults 100 International Units.

A deficiency of vitamin D in children causes rickets; and in malnourished women who have a number of pregnancies it can cause osteomalacia.

An excess of vitamin D occurs through overdosage of small children and can cause irritability, loss of appetite, loss of weight and occasionally death.

Vitamin E is associated with fertility in rats but in humans its use is still uncertain.

Vitamin K A deficiency of vitamin K in the human is associated with impaired clotting of the blood. The defieiency is unlikely to be caused by a low intake and is probably due to a defect in its use by the body.

The water soluble vitamins

Vitamin B is now known to be a collection of different vitamins.

1. *Vitamin B^1* or thiamine is necessary for the metabolism of glucose in the body and is probably of particular importance in the nourishment of nerve cells. A regular supply of this vitamin is needed because very little is stored in the body. It is present in a wide variety of foods including unrefined cereals, potatoes, green vegetables and milk. A deficiency of this vitamin is very rare in the United Kingdom unless a patient is not taking food. A deficiency,

is common in poorer countries particularly if rice or other cereals are refined. Beriberi is the result of deficiency.

2. There used to be a vitamin known as vitamin B^2 but is now known to be a group of vitamins of which the most important is riboflavine. Its source and use are similar to those of thiamine. Deficiency, which is rare in the United Kingdom, causes cracks at the corners of the mouth, a sore, red tongue and a dry, scaly skin.

3. *Nicotinic acid* is present in unrefined cereals and dairy products. Deficiency is most common in rice eating countries and causes pellagra. Exposed areas of the skin become pigmented and scaly, there is diarrhoea and there may be search mental symptoms including depression.

4. Vitamin B^6 is rather like vitamin E. its use is established in animals but in humans it is not yet understood. It is widely available in vegetables.

5. Vitamin B^{12} is present in meat and is necessary for the formation of blood cells. A deficiency occurs because it is not absorbed through the stomach wall and its lack causes pernicious anaemia. Replacement must be by repeated injections.

6. Folic acid is also necessary for the formation of blood cells and it is widely available in vegetables. A deficiency may occur in pregnant women and iron and folic acid may be given routinely during pregnancy to prevent anaemia.

Vitamin C or ascorbic acid is necessary for the healthy development of collagen in the body; this includes bones, teeth and the lining gof blood vessels. It is present in all fruits and vegetables but a good source is citrus fruits. The human adult needs about 30 mg a day and in the United Kingdom a quarter of this amount is normally supplied by potatoes. A deficiency of vitamin C causes scurvy and the disease is most commonly seen in elderly people who have an insufficient dietary intake.

5. Minerals

These, like vitamisn, are essential in the human diet for normal development and health; less, however, is known about many of them than about some vitamins.

1. *Sodium or salt.* All body fluids contain this mineral and the greater amount of it is in the extracellular fluid. The amount remains constant in the healthy adult. Sodium acts with potassium to stabilise the acid base balance. The daily intake necessary is about 1g but some people who like salty food may eat up to 10 g.

2. *Potassim* acts with sodium to keep a constant acid base balance in the body. Potassium is found mostly in intracellular fluid. Potassium is present in most foods that humans eat including fruit, vegetables and cereals. A deficiency is unlikely to be due to a low intake but to an excessive loss from the body as may occur in severe diarrhoea or while taking diuretics.

3. *Calcium* is present in the greatest quantity of all minerals in the body. Most of it is in the teeth and bones. The daily intake necessary is probably about 500 mg but it has been suggested that 1,000 mg could be necessary. It is present in large amounts in dairy foods particularly cheese and in 'hard' water and in many vegetables. A deficiency of calcium is seldom due to a lack in the dietary intake but to a failure of absorption as may occur in steatorrhoea; or to defective use in the body as may occur in diseases of the parathyroid.

4. *Phosphorusn* forms compounds with calcium in the bones and teeth. It also takes part in cell metabolism and reproduction. It is widely available in the diet and the body can deal with an excess by excretion in the stool or urine.

5. *Iron* is necessary in the body for the formation of haemoglobin. The daily intake needs to be about 10mg and probably up to 20mg in pregnant women. It is present in meat, bread and vegetables. A definicient intake causes one type of anaemia but in the United Kingdom this type of anaemia is more often due to an acute or chronic loss of blood than to a low intake of iron.

6. *Iodine* is vital to the body for the production of thyroxin by the thyroid gland. In most parts of the world it is present in the earth and water and vegetables in the diet have absorbed it. In areas where there is a shortage of iodine in the soil, humans may develop enlargement of the thyroid gland.

7. *Fluorine* occurs naturally in some soils and therefore in some water supplies. If is present in a quantity of about one part per million of water it lessens the incidence of dental caries. If present in amounts of 4 or 5 p.p.m. it can cause mottling of the teeth.

DIET FOR OBESITY

The problem of being overweight is largely one of more affluent, countries. It is usually caused by eating more than is necessary coupled with a sedentary way of life. Crash diets are of little use and a change in eating habits is necessary for the maintenance of permanent weight reduction.

During weight reduction the total intake of calories should be limited to 4,200kj (1,000 calories) a day and a steady weight loss of 0.5-1.0kg a week is sufficient.

A normal pattern of eating should be observed and the total calories divided foods should be omitted entirely:

Sugar, cakes, biscuits, sweet puddings

Alcohol

Fried foods

Chocolate, sweets, etc.

Jam, honey, marmalade, syrup, *etc.*

Dried fruits

Potato crisps

Sweet canned or bottled drinks

When the target weight has been reached the daily diet may be increased but the above foods are better omitted. A weekly check should be kept and a stricter diet started if the weight is increasing.

Diabetic Diets

A detailed description of a diabetic diet will not be given because physicians managing diabetes usually have their own methods of controlling diet.

The principles of any diabetic diet are the restriction of starches and sugars. The quantity allowed in the diet each day must be eaten and at regular intervals; this is particularly important if insulin is being used. In children it is more difficult to keep an exact control of these foods but it is best to encourage the diabetic child to take and early, responsible share in the management of his diet.

In all diabetic diets it is usual to aim at a daily fixed total calorie intake which may be about 7,500kj. This amount will vary with the sex, size and occupation of the patient. The diet is usually made up of about 210g of carbohydrate, 80g of protein and 70g of fat.

Carbohydrate is the nutrient which must be most carefully controlled and it is common to work out a system of dietary 'exchanges' based on the quantity of a food which contains 10g of carbohydrate.

The daily intake of milk will be controlled at about 3/4 pint and of butter at 1/2 oz.

It is usual to give the patient guidance about the following groups of foods which may also be controlled bu the 'exchange' system:

1. Foods which may be eaten in an unlimited quantity including tea and coffee without sugar and with milk form the daily allowance, clear soups, cheese, fish, meat, eggs and most vegetables.

2. Foods which may be eaten in moderation including all carbohydrate foods, fresh and dried fruit, pasta, thick soups, 'diabetic' foods and dry wines and sherry.

3. Foods to be avoided include sugar, sweets, jam, syrup, sweet puddings, ice-cream sweet, wines and sherry, spirits and liqueurs.

Equivalents for Use in Diabetic Diets

Bread: The equivalent to loz of bread (*i.e.* 15 grams of carbohydrate) is found in the following:

2 Ryvita or Vita-Weat.

3 Cream Crackers or Water Biscuits

3 Semi-sweet biscuits.

3/4 Cupful cornflakes or other breakfast cereal.

3 Tablespoons porridge.

1 Medium-sized potato (3 oz).

2 Tablespoons boiled rice, spaghetti or macaroni.

1/2 pint of milk.

Drinks: The following are equivalent to 20 grams of carbohydrate:

1 Glassful milk (7oz) and

2 Teaspoons Horlicks, Ovaltine or Bournvita.

2/3 Cupful fresh orange juice (4 oz) and 2 lumps or 2 teaspoon fuls of sugar.

Diabetic fruit squash and

4 Lumps or 4 teaspoons of sugar

1/2 Cup milk (3 oz) in tea or coffee and 1 oz bread (or equivalent).

Fruit: The following portions of fruit are equivalent to 10 grams of carbohydrate:

Apple, dessert	1 small.
Apple, stewed	1 $1\frac{1}{2}$ cups.
Apricots, dried	6 halves.
Apricots, fresh	2 medium.
Banana	1 small.
Cherries	10 large
Dates	2
Figs, dried	1 small
Figs, fresh	2 large
Gooseberries	6 large
Grapefruit	1 medium
Grapes	12
Greengages	4 medium
Melon	1 slice, 2 in thick
Orange	1 small
Orange Juice	2/3 cup
Peach	1 medium
Pear	1 medium
Pineapple, fresh	1 slice, 1 in thick
Plums, dessert	2 large

Plums, stewed	3 medium
Prunes	6 small
Raspberries	1 cup
Strawberries	1 cup
Tangerine	1 large

Foods to be voided in A Diabetic Diet

The following foods contain a high percentage of carbohydrate, and are therefore to be avoided by the diabetic: sugar, sweets, and chocolate; jam, marmalade, honey or syrup; puddings, cakes and pastries; biscuits (except ads equivalents to bread); sweetened fruit drinks and minerals.

Foods allowed at will in a Diabetic Diet

The following foods may be taken as desired by the diabetic: coffee, tea or soda water; clear broth, Bovril, Oxo or Marmite, and the following vegetables:

artichokes	chiocory	lettuce	radishes
asparagus	cucumber	marrow	rhubarb
broccoli	endive	mustard and	cress runner beasn
Brussels	French	mushrooms	sauerkraut
sprouts	beans		
cabbage	kale	onions	spinach
cauliflower	leeks	parsley	swedes
celery	lemons	pepper, green	tomatoes
			watercress

High Fibre Diet

This diet is increasinly used in constipation and in diverticulitis. It should include a large proportion of foods which are rich in fibres and relatively low in calories. These foods include:

Porridge and muesli

Bran which can be used in baking

Wholemeal flour and bread

Fresh and dried fruit

Vegetables and pulses

Unrefined rice

Gluten Free Diet

This diet is used in the management of coeliac disease and in other conditions in which the bowel is unable to deal with gluten. Gluten, a plant protein, is found in wheat, rye and barley. It is made of two parts which are glutenin and gliadin and it is the latter which is harmful. Flour can be produced which is free of gluten and this flour must be used in all baking for a patient who is unable to tolerate gluten. Very small amounts of gluten can be harmful and the diet must be strictly adhered to. All cereals which are not gluten free, *e.g.* cakes, biscuits, tinned foods, sauces, *etc.* which contain normal flour, must be excluded from the diet.

Low Saturated Fat Diet

This diet may be used in the management of diseases of the blood vessels and in multiple sclerosis. Fats to be avoided are those of animal origin and those which are solid at room temperature. Structurally the fats to be avoided are those that are saturated and the fats to be included in the diet are the mono-unsaturated or preferably the poly-unsaturated fats. The fats to be avoided are fat on meat, butter lard, cream, cheese and bacon. Milk should be skimmed and not more than two eggs should be eaten a week.

Sunflower seed oil is the best oil to use in the preparation of food and one of the varieties of poly-unsaturated margarine must be used instead of butter on bread and in baking.

Fatty fishes to be avoided include mackerel, herring and salmon; also all fish canned in oil such as sardines and tuna fish.

Low Residue And High Protein Diet

This diet may be used in the management of ulcertative colitis. All foods that are high in fibre content should be avoided. These include unrefined cereals, wholemeal bread, vegetables except potato, fruit and dried fruit and nuts. Fried food should also be avoided.

There should be an increased intake or lean meat, milk, fish, cheese (apart from cream cheese) eggs and refined cereals. Fruit juices and druit jellies should be included in the diet to ensure an adequate intake of vitamin C

Low Sodium Diet used Chiefly for Cardiac Failure

Avoid adding salt to food at meal times, and only *very* small quantities may be used in cooking.

The following food should be avoided: soups made from ham or salt meat; Oxo, Bovril; tinned and preserve meats; smoked and dried products such as ham and bacon; salt fish and offal (although heart and liver may be taken).

The patient should also avoid cheese; beetroot, celery

and spinach; puddings made with baking powder or soda; and anything made with self-raising flour.

He should not take meat sauces, pickles, slad cream or mayonnaise.

Low Fat Diet For Liver and Gallbladder Disease

Butter should be replaced by honey or golden syrup. No cheese. No nuts, chocolate or cocoa. Eggs are best avoided. No pastry or cakes, except small amounts of fatless sponge.

Lean meat is allowed: all fat should be carefully separated by the patient. Fat meat, ham, bacon and pork to be avoided. No suet. No sausages, liver, kidneys or offal. No fish or meat pastes.

Haddock, cod, whiting turbot, brill and plaice are allowed, but no other fish.

The patient should have skimmed milk.

Dietetics (Refers to). the study of food values.

Dietl's crises. Severe attacks of renal pain accompanied by scanty, bloodstained urine. Occurs in some cases of movable kidney probably due to kinking of the ureter.

Differential blood count. The determination of the proportion of each type of white cell in the blood, carried out by micro-scopical examination. Useful in diagnosis.

Digestion. Process of converting food into simple substances capable of absorption into the blood.

Digitalis. The foxglove; contains the active constituent from which digoxin and related substances are made. It slows, strengthens, regulates the heart beat and increases the cardiac output. It is indirectly a diuretic. It has a cumulative action. Vomiting, slow pulse, or 'coupling' of pulse in patient having this medication should be reported immediately.

Dilatation. Increase in size, enlargement. The operation of stretching.

Dilator. An instrument for dilating any narrow passage, as the rectum, uterus, urethra.

Diphtheria. A serious infectious disease, caused by corynebacterium diphtheriae. Any mucous membrane may be attacked but usually that of the throat or nose. A false, grey membrane develops in the pharynx. There is severe general malaise. An antitoxin is given and the patient kept at rest to avoid heart complications. *D. immunization*, a toxoid is injected prophylactically and all children from a year old should thus be protected against the disease.

Disease. A process which disturbs the structure or functions of the body.

Disinfectants. Agents which destroy micro-organisms; such as sunlight, heat, carbolic acid, sulphur dioxide, chlorine.

Disinfection. The thorough cleansing of an article with disinfectants in an attempt to destroy micro-organisms.

Dislocation. Displacement of the articular surface of a bone. Treatment, reduction under anaesthesia and immobilization. Congenital dislocation of the hip joint. The acetabulum is shallow and does not accommodate the head of the femur. The child has a wadding gait. Treatment is generally the Lorenz method by which after manipulation the hip is immobilized in plaster for many months. the thigh is abducted at a right angle to the trunk.

Dissection. A separation by cutting of parts, of the body.

Disseminated. Scattered throughout an organ or throughout the body. D. sclerosis, a chronic, degenerative disease of the nervous system. Also known as multiple sclerosis and insular sclerosis.

Doderlein's bacillus. Non-pathogenic bacillus present in secretions of the vagina.

Domette. A soft cotton and woollen fabric used for bandages.

Dominance. A factor present in the left cerebral hemisphere of humans, ehich makes people right - or left-handed. This lateral dominance is estblished early in childhood.

Dominant gene. A factor of inheritance that will manifest itself in the next generation.

Douche. A shower of water usually used to irrigate a cavity of the body. Hot douche 112° F (44 °C); cold douche 60 °f (16 °C).

Douglas's pouch. The peritoneal pouch between the back of the uterus and the front of the rectum.

Doyen's gag. A mouth gag much used by anaesthetists.

Doyen's speculum. a self-retaining speculum for keeping the incision widely open during abdominal operations.

Dracontiasis. Infestation by the guineaworm, comon parasite in tropical countries.

Drainage tubes. Tubes made of various materials which are inserted into operation wounds to allow materials such as blood to drain from the wound.

Drastic. Strong, severe.

Draught. A quantity of fluid to be taken at one time.

Drawsheet. A sheet so arranged that it can be removed easily from under a patient lying upon it.

Drinker's apparatus. One of the original mechanical

respirators, used to carry out artificial respiration when the respiratory muscles are paralysed, popularly known as the iron lung. The patient lies in a receptacle with his head only outside. A negative pressure is created in the receptacle by means of a suction pump; this draws air through the respiratory passages into the lungs. Now almost obsolete since the use of positive pressure ventilators.

Drip, intravenous. The administration into a vein of saline, plasma or blood.

Droplet infection. Droplets sprayed form a person's mouth, especially when talking, which infect other people.

Dropsy. Generalized oedema of tissues and fluid in the body cavities, as seen in cardiac failure.

Drug, Substance used as a medicine. *D. additction.* A dependence on drugs which is beyond the subject's control. *D. eruption.* Rash due to sensitivity to drug. D. reaction. General reaction to a drug. This may include fever, malaise, joint pains, rashes, jaundice, etc. D. resistance. Strains of micro-organisms resistant to the action of antibiotics.

Duchenne's disease. A progressive muscular atrophy, a disease of muscular tissue.

Ducrey's bacillus. The cause of soft sore or chancroid; a venereal disease. Small oval streptobacillus.

Duct. A tube or channel conveying the secretion of a gland generally lined by simple columnar or cuboidal epithelium.

Ductus. A duct; a little canal of body.

Dum-dum fever. Same as Kalazazar.

Dumping syndrome. The palpitations and gastric discomfort sometimes to felt by the patient after gastrecomy.

Duodenostomy. Surfical establishment of a communication between the duodenum and another structure.

Duodenum. The first 4 cm of the small intestine, beginning

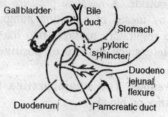

The duodenum

at the pyloric orifice of the stomach.

Dupuytren's contracture. A contracture of the palmar fascia affecting especially the ring and little fingers, which pulls them down into the palm so that they cannot be extended.

Dara mater. The outer membrane lining the interior of the cranium and spinal column.

Dwarf. Individual of stunted growth.

Dysaesthesia. The partial loss of feeling.

Dysarthria. Impairment of speech.

Dyschezia. Painful defaecation.

Dyschondroplasia. Multiple enchondromas. Cartilage is deposited in the shaft of some bone(s). Those affected which are often in the hands and feet, are short and deformed.

Dyscoria. Abnormality in the shape of the pupil.

Dyschromatopsia. Means loss of vision for colour.

Dysdiadokinesis. Inability to carry our rapid alternating movements, such as rotating the hands. A sign of cerebellar disease.

Dysentery. Inflammation of the large intestine. There are two kinds of dysentery, bacillary and amoebic; the former due to a bacillus, the latter to the *entamoeba histolytica.*

Dysfunction. Abnormal or impaired function.

Dyskinesia. Impairment of voluntary movement.

Dyslalia. Mechanical speech defect, cf. dysphasia.

Dyslexia. Difficulty in reading.

Dysmenorrhoea. Painful or difficult menstruation.

Dysorexia. A depraved or unnatural appetite.

Dyspareunia. Painful coitus.

Dyspepsia. Indigestion.

Dysphagia. Difficulty in swallowing.

Dysplasia. Difficulty in speaking.

Dysplasia, polyosteotic fibrous. Metabolic defect in the calcification of bone.

Dyspnoea. Difficult breathing.

Dystaxia. Difficulty in controlling voluntary movements. Mild ataxia.

Dystocia. A difficult labour (obstetric).

Dystrophy. Defective structure due to shortage of essential factors.

Dysuria. The painful micturition.

Ear. The organ of hearing. It consists of external, middle and internal ear.

The *external ear* comprises the auricle and external auditory canal, and is separated from the middle ear by the tympanic membrane.

The *middle ear* is an irregular cavity in the temporal bone. In front it communicates with the Eustachian tube which forms an open channel between the middle ear and the cavity of the nasopharynx. Behind, the middle ear opens into the mastoid antrum, and this in turn communicates with the mastoid cells. There are two openings into the inner ear, the foramen ovale and the foramen rotunda, both of which are covered with membrane. A string of tiny bones articulating with each other extend form the tym-panum to the *foramen ovale* of the internal ear. These bones are, from the tympanum— (1) malleus, (2) incus, (3) stapes.

The *internal ear* comprises (1) the organ of hearing or cochlea in which are the endings of the cochlear branch of the auditory nerve and (2) the organ of equilibrium or balance consisting of the three semicircular canals arranged at right angles to each other, and supplies by the vestibular branch of the auditory nerve.

Ecbolic. An agent used to stimulate the uterus and this acclerate the expulsion of the fetus, *e.g.* pituitary extract.

Ecchondroma. A tumour composed of cartilage.

Ecchymosis. A bruise; and effusion of blood under the skin.

ECG. *See* ELECTROCARDIOGRAM.

Echinococcus. One of the species of tape worm. In its adult stage it infests dogs. In its larval stage it produces hydatid cysts in man.

ECHO virus. Enteropathic cytopathic human orphan virus. *See* ADENOVIRUS. May cause benign lymphocytic meningitis and Bornholm disease.

Ectopic gestation. Pregnancy in which the fertilized ovum is not situated in the uterus. The ovum may lie in one of the Fallopian tubes or in the abdominal cavity. In coures of time the gestation sac is apt to rupture, causing profuse haemorrhage into the abdominal cavity and necessitating immediate operation.

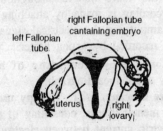

Ectopic gestation: fertilized ovum in right Fallopian tube.

Eczema. Inflammation of the skin, acute or chronic. There is redness and vesicles may appear which weep and form crusts.

Elastoplast bandage. An adhesive bandage containing zinc oxide.

Elation. A happy and exalted state of mind.

Elbow. The joint between the arm and forearm formed by the humers above, and the radius and ulna below.

Electra complex. Excessive love for a father by a daughter who hates her mother. Named after Electra in Greek mythology.

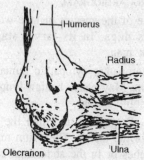

The elbow joint

Electrocardiogram. ECG. Recording of electrical events occurring in the heart muscle throughout the cardiac cycle. The recording is made by attaching electrodes to the skin and amplifying the electrical signal. The oscilations may be recorded by a pen writer.

Electrocardiophonography. Recording of heart sounds electrically by a phonocardiograph.

Electroconvulsive therapy. ECT. Therapy used especially in depressive mental illness, consisting of passing a low amperage electric current between electrodes placed on the side of the head. The reaction is modified by general anaesthesia and muscle relaxant drugs given before the shock treatment.

Electro-encephalography. Recording of electric currents resulting from cerebral activity.

Electromyography. EMG. The recording of electrical events occurring in muscle.

Electron. A negatively charged atomic particle. E. microscopy. The use of electrons instead of light to visualize microscopic objects. The apparatus is complex but allows very much greater resolution to be obtained and therefore more details to be seen.

Electroretinogram. Recording of electrical variations in the retina on exposure to light.

Elephantiasis or **filariasis.** A parasitic disease of the lymphatic vessels causing great enlargement of the limb or limbs affected (usually the leg). It is chronic and the skin thickens until it somewhat resembles an elephant's hide. The parasite is the Filaria.

Elixir. A term some times applied to certain preparation of drugs having a sweet taste.

Emasculation. Castration of the male.

Embolectomy. Removal of an embolus.

Embolism. Obstruction of blood vessel, usually an artery by a body, *e.g.* portion of thrombus, fat cells, air transported in the bloodstream. If the embolus is large enough to block completely any of the valvular orifices of the right side of the heart, sudden death is the result: if small enough to pass through the right side of the heart, the embolus may be arrested somewhere in the pulmonary artery or in one of its subdivisions, giving rise to an infact of the lung, with symptoms of intense sudden pain in the chest, coughing of blood, and great distress. In certain cases of valvular disease of the heart, pieces of clot formed upon the affected value break off and are carried away in the bloodstream. When such an embolus reaches an artery too small for it, an embolism results, with symptoms according to the organ affected. Embolism of an artery of the brain may result in immediate death or in paralysis.

Embolus. A blood clot or other foreign body in the bloodstream.

Embrocation. A lotion for rubbing on the skin.

Embryo. Animal in process of development from the fertilized ovum.

Embryology. Science of the development of the embryo.

Embryotome. An instrument for destroying any part of the child during birth for the purpose of facilitating delivery.

Emetic. Any means used to produce vomiting. Tickling the throat with a feather; specified preparations of ipecacuanha. Apomorphine, given hypodermically.

Empyema. A collection of pus in a cavity, most commonly referring to the pleural cavity. The term is also used for collections of pus in the maxillary antrum, frontal sinus, and other cavities.

Encephalitis. Inflammation of the brain. *See* MENINGITIS. *E. lethargica.* Encephalitis associated with profound disturbance of sleep rhythm.

Endocervicitis. Inflammation of the mucouc membrane lining the canal of the cervix uteri.

Endocolpitis, Inflammation of inner coat of the vagina.

Endocrine. the term used in describing the ductless glans giving rise to an internal secretion. The endocrines are—suprarenals, thymus, thyroid, parathyroids, pituitarty, pancreas, ovaries, and testicles. The pancreas acts as both an endocrine organ and for the secretion of digestive juices. It therefore also has ducts.

Endocrinology. Science of the endocrine glands.

Endoderm. Germ layer of embryo composed, as is mesoderm, of cells which have migrated from the surface to the interior of the embryo during gastrulation, and from which the alimentary tract is largely derived.

Endogenous. Produced with in the body *e.g.* endogenous inection.

Endolymph. Fluid of the membranous labyrinth of the ear.

Endometrioma. Tumour, from tissue like that of the endometrium but found outside it in myometrium, ovary, uterine ligaments, rectovaginal septum, peritoneum, caecum, pelvic colon, umbilicus and laparotomy scars.

Endoscope. An instrument for the inspection of the interior of a hollow organ.

Endosteoma. Tumour within a bone cavity.

Endosteum, The medullary membrane of bone. *See* BONE.

Endothelioma. A malignant growth originating in endothelium.

Endothelium. The lining membrane of series cavities, blood vessels and lymphaties.

Enema. An injection into the bowel. it can be given with a rectal tube and funnel but rectal suppositories and disposable enemas are replacing funnel.

Engagement of head. Descent of fetal head into the cavity of the pelvis, Normally occurs two to four weeks before term in the primigravida but in multigravida may not occur until labour.

Engorgement. Vascular congestion.

Enophthalmos. Recession of the eyeball into the orbit.

Enostosis. A tumour in a bone.

Enteroviruses. Viruses belonging to the pico RNA virus group. Es. enter the body by the alimentary tract and comprise the three polio viruses, the Coxsackie virus causing Born-holm disease and the ECHO viruses causing aseptic meningitis.

Epiloia. Tuberous sclerosis. Inherited defect characterized by sebaceous adenoma of the face, multiple gliomas in the brain and tumours of the heart, kidneys and retina. Fits are the earliest signs of the disease and mental deficiency usually follows.

Epimenorrhoea. Menstrual periods of frequent recurrence.

Epinephrectomy. Excision of suprarenal gland.

Epineurium. The sheath of nerve.

Epiphora. An excessive flow of tears.

Epiphysis. The separately ossified end of growing bone separated from the shaft diaphysis, by a cartilaginous plate (epiphyseal plate). When growth is completed the epiphysis and diaphysis fuse.

Epiphysitis. Inflammation of an epiphysis.

Epiplocele. A hernia containing omentum.

Epiploon. The omentum.

Erb's paralysis. The muscles of the upper arm are paralysed due to a lesion of the fifth and sixth cervical nerve roots. May result from excessive traction on the arm during labour. It hangs limply, rotated internally from the shoulder, elbow extended, forearm pronated and palm of hand turned outwards.

Erectile tissue. Specialized vascular tissue which becomes, rigid when filled with blood. *e.g.* penis.

Eretor. A muscle which raises a part.

Erepsin. A ferment of the succus entericus (secretion of the small intestines). It completes the digestion of the protein.

Ergograph. An instrument for recording the amount of work done by mucular action.

Ergosterol. A sterol found in fats and present in the skin which is converted into vitamin D by irradiation with ultraviolet light.

Erythema. Red skin, due to vasodilatation in the dermis. *E. multiforme.* Lesions consisting of raised red lesions of varying size and shape which may blister. The cause is unknown but it may represent an abnormal immune response. *E. nodosum.* Red tender skin nodules on the legs which may occur in certain conditions such as tuberculosis and sarcoidosis.

Esbach's albuminometer. A graduated tube used to estimate the quantity of albumin in urine.

Eschar. A dry healing scab on a wound; generally the result of the use of caustic. Also the mortified part in dry gangrene.

Esmarch's bandage. An india-rubber bandage which is tightly applied to the limb, beginning at the extremity, and when it has reached above the point of operation a stout tube is wound round the limb and fastened. This provides a bloodless surgical field.

Ethnology. The science of the races of mankind.

Eustachian tube. The canal from the throat to the ear.

Euthanasia. A planned and painless death procured by the use of drugs.

Eutocia, Eeasy labour (obstetric).

Eve's method. A method of artificial respiration. By placing the patient in a special rocking apparatus, the diaphragm is forced up and down.

Ewing's tumour. Malignant tumour of bone occurring in young adults.

Exenteration. Removal of all contents. *E. of orbit.*1 Removal of all contents of the bony orbit. *E. of pelvis.* Removal of pelvic contents and transplantations of ureters into the sigmoid colon.

Exfoliation. Excessive loss of superficial layers of skin in thin flakes.

Exhibitionism. Behaving in a way to attract attention and term used in psychiatry for sex perversion such as indecent exposure.

Exhumation. Disinterment of the body.

Exotoxin. Toxin released from exterior of an organism, cf. endotoxin.

Expectorant. A drug which increases expectoration.

Expectoration. The coughing up of sputum.

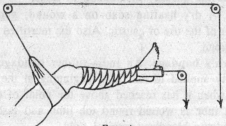

Extension apparatus

Exploration. Operative surgical investigation.

Expression. (1) The act of expulsion (2) Facial appearance.

Exsanguinate. To make bloodless.

Extension. (1) A certain pull or weight applied to a fractured, dislocated, or contracted limb to keep it straight. There are two methods, (a) Skin traction applied as follows: A long piece of strapping, about 2 in wide, with a stirrup, consisting of a square piece of wood the same width as that of the foot at the ankle, and with a hole in the middle, is required; also some short narrower pieces of strapping. To apply it, the stirrup should be about 4 in below the foot, and the strapping attached to it should be carried up the inside the outside of the leg well above the knee: the short pieces of strapping are put round the leg from the ankle to below the knee. A knotted piece of cord is passed through the hole in the wood over a pulley at the foot of the bed. Weights are attached to the cord, the number varying according to the age of the patient and condition for which it is applied. For a fractured femur $\frac{1}{7}$ of the body weight is usually satisfactory.

The foot of the bed should be slightly raised (b) Skeletal traction, a Steinmann's pin or Kirschner wire is passed through the lower fragment of the bone or an ice-tong caliper may be inserted. (2) The straightening of a flexed limb or part.

Extensor. A muscle which extends a part.

External version. A method of changing the lie or presentation of the fetus by manipulation of the uterus through the abdominal wall.

Extracellular fluid. That part of the body fluid not contained in cells nor the blood.

Extract. Concentrated preparation of a drug: it may be in a liquid or solid form, *e.g.* extract of cascara.

Extrapyramidal. Motor nerve tracts and associated centres which do not directly communicate with the main motor pathway (pyramidal tract). It is a very complex system with many functions, one of which is to regulate muscle tone.

Extrasystoles. Systolic contraction of the heart the impulse for which originates in a focus other than the sinuatrial node, and is therefore outside the normal chain of events in the cardiac cycle.

Extra-Uterine gestation. Pregnancy outside the uterus.

Extravasation. Escape of fluid from its proper channel into surrounding tissue.

Extrovert. Thinking of things other than one-self. The op-

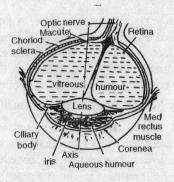

Horizontal section of right eye

posite kind of temperament to introvert.

Exudation. Oozing; slow escape of liqued.

Eye. The organ of vision. illustration.

Eye-strain. Headache due to effort required to focus on
near objects when the refractive properties of the lens are
defective.

F

Facies. Facial expression particularly applied to expressions which are diagnostic of certain conditions, *e.g.* abdominal facies, adenoid facies.

Faecal. Relating to the faeces.

Faeces. The discharge from the bowels. Common abnormalities to be noted are *Colour*— Black may indicate the presence of altered blood or the patient may be taking iron. Green stools occur in enteritis. Clay-coloured stools in jaundice. *Consistency* — Loose watery stools occur in diarrhoea, hard dry stols in constipation. Foreign bodies such as worms may be present. Unaltered blood may be due to haemorrhoids. Mucus and blood may be due to coliteis or intussusception.

Fallopian tubes. Two trumpet-like canals, about 7.5 cm long, passing from the overies to the uterus.

Fallot's tetralogy. A group of congenital heart defects consisting of dextraposition of the aorta, right ventricle hypertrophy, intraventricular septal defect and stenosis of the pulmonary artery.

Fantus test. Test for the presence of chloride in the urine.

Farinaceous. Containing flour or grain. Farinaceous diet consists of milk puddings, gruel, bread, and other starchy foods.

Fascia. A fibrous structure separating one compartment of the body from another, or one muscle from another.

Fat. An organic compound which is a desirable constituent of human diet. Mother's milk contains about 4 per cent of fat in finely divided globules. Cow's milk contains about 4-6 per cent of tat. Cream contains up to 20 per cent.

Fatigue. Tiredness.

Fatty degeneration. Term applied to the appearance of certain cells which as a result of damage take on an appearance of having droplets of fat in their cytoplasm.

Fehling's solution. Sulphate of copper and potassium hydrate are the chief ingredients; the solution was used as a test for sugar in the urine.

Felon. A whitlow. An inflammation of the finger near the nail.

Felty's syndrome. A kind of rheumatoid arthritis and associated with leucopenia and splenomegaly.

Female. Applied to the sex that bears young.

Femoral artery. The artery of the thigh, from the groin to the knee.

Femoral canal. The small canal internal to the femoral vein. the site of femoral hernia.

Femur. The thigh bone.

Fertility. Ability to produce young.

Fertilization. Union of male and female germ cells whereby reproduction takes place.

Fester. Inflammation with collection of pus.

Festination. Propulsive giat as in Parkinsonism.

Fetishism. The worship of an inanimate object which symbolizes a loved person.

Fetus. The unborn child. Formerly frequently spelt foetus.

Fetus papyraceus. Fetus which has been retained within the uterus for months after its death, and has undergone a kind of natural mummification.

Fever. A rise in body temperature above normal. There is generally a quick pulse, lassitude, often delirium, and inhibition of the secretory glands. The nursery treament is rest, freedom from chills, and light nourishing diet with abundant fluids.

Fibroelastosis. Rare disorder affecting the heart. Excess collagen and elastin form under the endocardium.

Fibroid. A tumour composed of fibrous and muscular tissue.

Fibromyoma. A tumour composed of mixed muscular and fibrous tissue. Especially common in the uterus, and commonly spoken of as 'fibroids'.

Fibrosis. Deposition of fibrous connective tissue usually occurring in regions which have been damaged by some trauma.

Finger. One of the digits of the hand.

FIRST AID

The AIMS of first aid are;

1. To save life.

2. To prevent the injury and the effects of the injury getting worse.

3. To get a live patient to hospital or into other medical care.

4. To reduce the anxiety of the patient.

First aid may be carried out by a doctor but it can also be carried out effectively by anybody trained in the art of giving first aid and practised in applying it.

ALCOHOL should never be given.

NO DRINKS should be given to any patient apart from the conscious severely burned adult.

Priorities

The first aider must identify and treat urgently all life-threatening conditions. To this end the following question should be asked about each casualty and answered as rapidly and accurately as possible in order that the appropriate steps may be instigated :

1. Should the patient be removed from a position of danger such as a live source of electricity?

2. Is the patient breathing or not breathing ? The brain can live for only about four minutes without a supply of oxygen reaching it in the blood. Do not waste time splinting or bandaging a patient who is not breathing. A hospital can treat a live casualty but not a dead one.

3. Is the patient bleeding severely ? Both internal and external bleeding need to be recognized and immediate attention paid to stopping any visible bleeding; a casualty with internal bleeding needs urgent transfer to hospital.

4. It the patient conscious or unconscious ? Diagnosing the cause of unconsciousness is not of immeditae concern to the first aider but the correct positioning of the patient will save life and must be practised by all those who study first aid.

Removing the Patient From A Position of Danger

This may involve turning off an electric supply with a well-insulated device or dragging the patient out of water. A casualty trapped in a car should be left until a doctor and, if possible, the fire brigade arrive. The first aider should only attempt to carry out this manoeuver if the car is on fire. If you are dragging a casualty out of water, artificial respiration can and should be started before you have the patient in an ideal place and position.

Is the Patient Breathing?

If the casualty is not breathing artificial respiration should be started with the minimum dealy. The following measures should be carried out as rapidly as possible because there is no time to waste.

a. Put the casualty flat on his back, arch his neck and lift his lower jaw upwards and forwards. This will lift his tongue away from the back of his throat and provide an airway (Figs. 53 & 54).

b. Clear the mouth of any debris including pieces of food and false teeth.

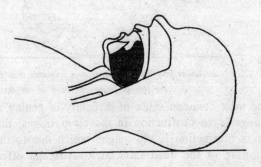

The tongue blocking the throat of an unconscious patient

c. Keeping the jaw in the correct position with one hand under the patient's chin, take a deep breath in. Place your pen mouth firmaly over the patient's nose while keeping his mouth shut with upward pressure under his chin. Breathe out steadily and firmly until you see the patient's chest rise. Lift your head, turn it to one side, take a deep breath in and repeat the manoeuver (Figs. 55 & 56). If mouth-to-nose respiration is impossible mouth-to-mouth respiration should be carried on.

d. Artificial respiration should be continued until either the patient breathes spontaneously, a doctor says that he is dead, or if a doctor is not available it should be continued for at least an hour.

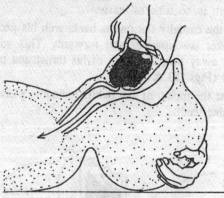

the lower jaw lifted upwards and forwards thus lifting the tongue from the back of the throat.

The most common cause of difficulty in getting air into the lungs is an obstruction in the air passages; the most common obstruction is the tongue which due to the mal-positioning of the head falls backwards and effectively blocks the passage at the back of the nose and mouth. Have a quick look in the mouth to make sure that no further debris has appeared and then lift the lower jaw and pull it. Forward Correct the extension of the neck by putting one hand under the nape of the neck and pulling the head backward with the other hand. Continue mouth-to-nose or mouth-to-mouth respiration.

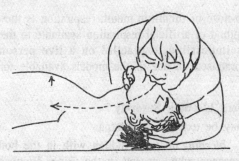

Mouth-to-nose respiration. The chest of the casualty rises as it fills with air.

If you are using this method of artificial respiration on a child, care must be taken in the amount of air blown into the lungs. The chest must be watched constantly because damage can be done to the lungs by over-vigorous inflation. If the patient is a small child it is usually easier for the first aider to put his mouth over the child's nose and mouth.

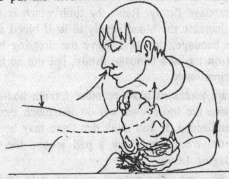

Operator takes away his mouth and breathes in himself. The chest of the casualty falls on expiration.

Vomiting may occur while artificial respiration is being carried out. The patient's head should be turned immediately to one side and the mouth rapidly cleaned out before artificial respiration is continued.

Mouth-to-nose or mouth-to-mouth respiration is the most effective method of artificial respiration available to the first aider. It is impossible to practise on a live person but should be practised on one of the models available for this purpose.

Is the Patient bleeding Severely ?

Bleeding may be external or interna.

External bleeding may be hidden with in the body or show its presence when passed in the urine, coughed up, etc. Internal bleeding may be severe around a fracture particularly that of the femur or thigh bone.

The diagnosis of severe bleeding must be made quickly because the loss of a litre of blood is serious.

External bleeding will be seen if looked for. Press on the area from which the blood is coming. A sterile pad is best but a bare hand is better than nothing. Put a pad over the area and bandage firmly. Raise the limb which is injured in order to decrease the blood supply to it. If blood appears through the bandage, do not remove the dressing but put another pad on top and bandage firmly, but not so tight as to cut off circulation.

If there are pieces of glass or other foreign bodies in a wound remove the loose ones but do not touch those that are firmly embedded. If you think that there may be a fracture under the wound build up a pad around the wound before bandaging firmly.

Internal bleeding. The patient will be pale, cold and sweating. There may be swelling from an injury such as a fractured femur. No time should be lost trying to make an accurate diagnosis. The casualty should be sent to hospital because he will need replacement of the blood lost as well as treatment of his injuries.

Is the Patient Conscious or Unconscious?

A conscious patient makes some effort to answer a question or obey a command.

If a casualty is breathing but unconscious he should be put in the unconscious position (Fig. 57). Clear any debris from the patient's mouth. Turn the patient on to his front and his face towards you. Bend his leg, nearest to you, at the knee and bring it towards you over the other leg. Bend the arm nearest to you, at the elbow and bring the forearm towards you and let it rest on the ground parallel to the casualty's face. Finally lift his chin upwards. If possible arrange the casualty so that he has a slight head down tip.

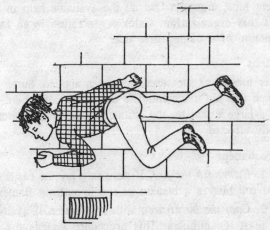

The unconscious position

An unconscious patient must not be left alone. A constant watch must be kept to make sure that he continues to breathe, does not choke and is gently controlled if he becomes restless.

If patient is unconscious and not breathing artificial

respiration must be initiated immediately. If he starts breathing but remains unconscious he must then be put in the unconscious position.

ALL CASUALTIES who have needed treatment for FAILURE TO BREATHE or for UNCONSCIOUSNESS must be seen by a doctor at a hospital.

Organization

At some point while dealing with a number of casualties who have life-threatening conditions you must also get an estimate of the total number of casualties and send somebody to arrange for ambulances and a doctor if possible. you will need to decide which patients need hospital treatment most urgently. Use all the available help in carrying out this organization. Calm organization is an important function of a trained first aider.

Burns

After life-saving measures have been applied, burns must be given first aid treatment. The seriousness of a burn depends to a large extent on the amount of the surface area of the body affected.

Treatement

1. *Extinguish the fire.* If necessary lay the casualty down and roll him in a blanket or rog to put out flames.

2. *Cool the burnt area* with cold water, if available, for at least ten minutes. This procedure lessens the damage done to the body tissues by the burn and also relieves the pain.

3. *Cover the burnt area.* Use a sterile dressing if possible; if such dressings are not avilable use any clean pieces of cloth.

DO NOT USE ANY OINTMENT OR LOTION.

DO NOT BURST ANY BLISTERS.

Keep the casualty lying down until he reaches hospital. A large amount of fluid is lost from burnt areas and to remedy this loss conscious adult casualties should be given frequent small drinks of liquid.

DO NOT GIVE ALCOHOL

Burns of the eye should be washed under gently running water for at least ten minutes and then covered with a clean dry dressing until medical help can be obtained.

A SEVERELY BURNT PATIENT NEEDS QUIET, CALM HANDLING AND A GREAT DEAL OF REASSURANCE.

Fractures and Dislocations

A fracture is any break or crack in a bone. A fracture may be either closed or open.

1. *A clsoed fracture.* The skin is intact over the area of the fracture.

2. *An open fracture.* The skin is broken over the area of the fracture. This is important because germs can enter and cause infection.

A dislocation is the disruption of a joint and occurs most commonly at the shoulder joint and the jaw. A gain this may be closed or open.

Diagnosis of a fracture or dislocation can only be made conclusively by an x-ray. This is beyound the scope of the first aider but the following signs are suggestive.

1. History of a fall or other violent injury.

2. Pain.

3. Tenderness on examination.

4. Swelling.

5. Loss of power.

6. Deformity.

Treatment

Alway remember that the fracture of a large bone such as the femur can be a major cause of blood loss and a blood transfusion may be the most urgent treatment. Never waste time on elaborate splinting; concentrate on getting a live patient to hospital but remember the following principles:

1. A clsoed fracture must never become an open fracture through   careless handling.

2. An open fracture must be covered to prevent infection.

3. The fracture must be prevented from getting worse during the journey to hospital.

4. Never cause the casualty greater pain during the diagnosis or treatment. The fractured area will be very tender and must be handled with great care.

5. No attempt must be made to restore a dislocated joint to its normal position.

The two basic principles to be observed in the treatment of all fractures and dislocation are:

1. Immobilization to increase the comfort of the patient and prevent the injury getting worse.

2. Speedy removal to hospital for expert diagnosis and treatment.

If you are in doubt about the diagnosis of a fracture treat the injury as a fracture.

If one arm or one leg is fractured the uninjured limb can be used as a standard of normality and the injured limb compared with it for size and shape. Elaborate splinting is unnecessary and may do more harm than good by causing undue movement of the casualty and delaying his removal to hospital.

Basic Priniples of Splinting

1. The site of the fracture must be immobilized together with the joint above and below it.

2. The natural contours of the body should be levelled out by soft padding or a rolled up woollen scarf, rags, etc.

3. No bandages should be put on so tightly that the blood circulation is hindered.

Fractures of the shoulder blade and upper arm: Loose padding should be put between the arm and the body. The chest can be used as a splint and the arm placed in the most comfortable position against it—usually with the elbow bent and the forearm in a sling. This position immobilizes both the shoulder and elbow joints.

Fractures of the elbow and lower arm: Padding should be placed between the arm and the body but the elbow should not be bent. The casualty will usually be more comfortable lying on a stretcher with the injured arm tied gently to the side of his body.

Fractures of the wrist and hand: The elbow can be bent and a sling used to keep the forearm and hand immobilized against the front of the chest.

Fractures of the thigh bone or femur: These are serious injuries because of the large amount of blood that can be lost around the site of the fracture. It is important that the casualty should be sent to hospital as soon as possible. Lay the casualty flat on a stretcher. Put padding between the knees, ankles and contours of the legs. Gentleness is important. Tie the feet together with a figure of eight bandage (Fig. 58). Tie the knees together and place bandages around both legs above and below the fracture. Always remember

that the casualty will be severely ill with this fracture and
be gentle, calm and reassuring.

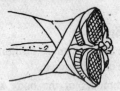

Figure of eight bandage for lower limb fracture

Fractures below the knee: Remember that in all fractures
of the shin bone or tibia the injury is likely to be or to become an open fracture. If one leg is fractured the sound leg
may be used as a splint for the injured one. Lay the casualty flat. Place padding between the thigs, knees and ankles.
Tie the feet together with a figure of eight bandage. Tie the
knees together and both legs together with bandages above
and below the fracture.

If both legs are fractured the injury is a very severe one.
If possible two long splints should be used, one on each
side of the body, long enough to reach from the armpits to
beyond the feet. If such splints are not available one splint
should be used from the level of the groin to beyond the
feet and put between the two legs. Padding should be
placed between the long splints or the shorter splint and the
contours of the body and around the knees and ankles. The
feet should be tied together with a figure of eight bandage.
Tie the knees together and put bandages around both legs
and the splints above and below the levels of the fractures.
If two long splints are being used additional bandages
should be put around the hips and chest.

Fractures of the jaw: Bandaging is unneccessary. If both
sides of the jaw are fractured passage of air into the lungs

may be affected. An unconscious casualty should be put in the unconscious position. A conscious casualty should be in a sitting position with the head tilted slightly forward. The casualty must be taken to hospital.

Fracture of the hip bone or pelves: This can be a serious injury depending on the amount of damage that is done inside the body. The casualty must be put on his back on a stretcher. Put padding between his knees and ankles. Tie his feet together with a figure of the eight bandage. Warn the casualty not to pass water on his way to hospital.

Fracture of the spine: This can be a very serious injury and be both life-threatening and the cause of paralysis below the site of the fracture. Send for help, a stretcher and an ambulance.

No attempt should be made to move the casualty unitl at least four and preferably five people are present. The movement of the casualty on to a stretcher is a job for an expert because the position of the spine must not be changed at any time during the manoeuvre. Minor flexion or bending forward of the spine is the most dangerous change of position because it can compress the spinal cord and cause irreversible damage to the nerves below the level of the fracture.

Dislocations: Any dislocation is a very painful and frightening injury and the casualty needs ressurance and calm treatment.

No attempt must be made to restore the joint to its normal position. The injured area must be supported in the position which is most comfortable for the casualty. The casualty must be taken to hospital.

Poisoning

Poisoning is hazard that should be prevented rather than treated. There are so many poisonous substances now in general use that it is impracticable to give the treatment of each one. A general outline will be given.

ALWAYS KEEP A CONTAINER FROM WHICH THE POISON IS BELIEVED TO HAVE BEEN TAKEN AND SEND IT TO HOSIPITAL WITH THE PATIENT.

If the patient is not breathing artificial respiration must be given. When the patient starts breathing put him in the unconscious position. Send him to hospital.

If the casualty is conscious but shows signs of burning in or around the mouth send him urgently to hospital and do not make him vomit.

If the casualty is conscious and shows no signs of burning in or around his mouth make him vomit. This can usually be achieved by putting your finger down the back of his throat. If you are trying to make a child vomit put a spoon handle down the back of his throat and not your finger. After he has vomited give him at least a litre of water, milk, weak tea or coffee while waiting for him to be taken to hospital or on the way.

Miscellaneous mishaps

Foreign bodies in the eye: A loose foreign body in the eye may be moved by rapid blinking of the eye or by pulling the upper lid outwards and downwards over the lower lid. No attempt should be made to remove a foreign body forcibly even if it can be clearly seen. A pad should be put over the eye and medical help obtained.

Foreign bodies in the nose and ear: These are usually self-inflicted accidents by small children. The presence of the foreign body may only be suspected by the observation of a one sided blood or pus stained discharge. No attempt should be made to remove the object and medical advice should be obtained.

Nose Bleeds: A nose bleed may follow an injury to the nose and is sometimes associated with a fracture. More often a nose bleed occurs spontaneously. The casualty should then be made to sit leaning slightly forwards and hold a pad of handkerchief or soft paper firmly around the end of his nose. Sniffing must be discouraged and the pad should be held in place for ten minutes after the bleeding has stopped.

Snake Bites: In the United Kingdom the only poisonous snake is the adder. Its bite is seldom dangerous or fatal but the anxiety is produces is very great. The casualty should be lain down and the bitten limb raised. No attempt should be made to cut or suck the bite. The casualty should be taken to hospital.

In parts of the world where snake bites can be fatal the same initial treatment should be given and transport to hospital arranged as speedily as possible. It may be helpful if the species of the snake can be identified so that appropriate treatment can be given.

First intention. A surgical term for aseptic healing of a wound by bringing the edges directly together.

First stage. The act of parturition from the first pains to full dilatation of the cervix.

Fistula. Any unnatural passage communicating with two epithelialized surfaces. *Fistula in ano*, anal fistula: any sinus connected with the anus and therefore discharging faeces. See ISCHIO-RECTAL ABSCESS. FAECAL FISTULA. A communication between the bowel and the surface; this may be a complication of an abdominal operation. General peritonitis seldom occurs, as track of the discharge from bowel to surface becomes walled off by adhesions. They tend to close spontaneously, but take some weeks. Internal fistula is an artificial opening between two viscera— *e.g.* (1) biliary fistula, between the gall bladder and intestine. (2) A visico-vaginal F., A communication between the bladder and the vagina; this may be a complication of an extensive operation on the female generative organs.

Fit. Convulsion, usually with loss of consciousness.

Flap. A piece of skin cut to fold over the stump in operation for amputation.

Flatfoot, Flattening or total loss of arches of the foot. It then rests completely on the ground, giving characteristic appearance and walk.

Flatulence. gas in the alimentary canal, usually refers to the stomach. It may be produced by simply swallowing air or by the fermentation of food. Carminatives give relief.

Flatus. Gas in the alimentary canal, usually refers to the bowel. It may be relieved by passing a flatus tube.

Flea. The human flea is *Pulex irritans*. It is without wings and sucks blood, giving rise to irritation and sepsis.

Flexion. Being bent; the opposite of extension.

Flexner bacillus. One of the Shigella group of bacteria causing bacillary dysentery.

Flexor. A muscle which causes flexion.

Flexure. A bend. A curvature of an organ, e.g. Hepatic f. Bend of the colon beneath the liver.

Floating ribs. The two lower pairs of ribs not articulating with sternum.

Flooding. Excessive bleeding from the uterus.

Fluke. Any of the trematode class of worm.

Fluorescein. A coal-tar derivative which stains cornea a vivid green if there is any loss of surface epithelium - e.g. in an abrasion or ulcer.

Flying squad. Emergency obstetric unit which can travel rapidly to domiciliary cases of complicated labour.

Foetor. Strong unpleasant smell.

Folic acid. Pteroyl-glutamic acid, part of the vitamin B complex found in liver, yeast, spinach, etc. Essential for blood formation.

Follicle. A minute bag containing some secretion.

Follicle stimulating hormone. ESH. Harmone secreted by the anterior lobe of the pituitary gland. In the female it stimulates the growth of overian follicles and the production of oestrogens. In the male it promotes the development of spermatozoa in the testis.

Follicular tonsillitis. Pus in the follicles of the tonsils. The tonsils are red and sowllen and covered with small yelow spots.

Fomentations. Lint or fannel wrung out in some boiling fluid and applied for the alleviation of pain. It must be wrung out throughly and shaken to allow escape of steam and applied as hot as can be borne; cover lint with a slightly larger piece of jaconet and then a still larger piece of wool, and bandage whole securely.

Fomites. Articles of clothing or bedding which have been in contact with a patient ill with a contagious disease.

Fontanelle. A soft space in the skull of an infact before the skull has completely ossified. The anterior fontanelle, or bregma, is where the coronal, frontal and sagittal sutures meet. The posterior fontanelle is where the lambdoid and sgittal sutures meet. The anterior fontanelle is normally

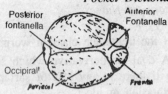

The fontanelles

closed by 2 years of age and delay in closure is a sign
of rickets.

Food poisoning. Diarrhoea and/or vomiting from eating infected food. Symptoms may be caused by the preformed
toxins, of *Staphylococcus aureus* or *Clostridium welchii*
or from infection by organisms of the *salmonella group*
or rarely by *botulinus toxin*. Infected foods are usually
meat products or confectionery containing eggs, which
have been allowed to remain in warm rooms. Another
source of infection may be the unwashed hands of those
handling food.

Foot. That part of the leg below the ankle.

Foot and mouth disease. Virus disease well-known in cattle. It occasionally affects man, causing blistering of the
buccal mucoccsa and similar lesions on the hands and
feet, especially round the nails.

Foot drop. Inability to keep a foot bent at right angles with
the leg. The toes and foot drop and walking becomes difficult. Caused by pressure of bedclothes, or inadequate
support to under side of foot when leg is in a splint for
a long time, or from paralysis of the muscles which
produce dorsiflexion of the ankle.

Foramen. An opening *F. magnum.* Opening in the back of
the skull through which the spinal cord passes. *F. ovale.*
Opening between the right and left atria in the fetus
which allows oxygenated venous blood from the placenta
to pass into the left side of the heart thus by-passing the

pulmonary circulation. It normally closes at birth. *Optic f.*, where the optic nerve enters the skull.

Forceps. Surgical pincers used for lifting and moving instead of using the fingers.

Forebrain. Cerebrum.

Forensic medicine. Medicine in so far as it has to do with the law.

Formaldehyde. A powerful antiseptic. Its gas is used to disinfect unoccupied rooms.

Fossa. Little depressions of the body, such as *fossa lacrimalis*, the hollow of the frontal bone, which holds the lacrimal gland. *Iliac fosae.* Concavities of the iliac bones of the pelvis.

Fothergill's operation. Repair of the anterior and posterior vaginal walls and amputation of the cervix.

Fourchette. A thin fold of skin behind the vulva.

Fractional test meal, Performed to examine the gastric contents and to estimate the rate of emptying of the stomach. A substance is given to stimulate the gastric glands and the resultant secretion of hydrochloric acid is estimated.

Fracture. A break in a bone. The symptoms are pain, swelling, deformity, loss of function, unnatural mobility, shortening, crepitus. A fracture may be: (1) *Simple* or *closed*, not connected with an external wound. (2) *Compound* or *open*, communicating with the surface. (3) *Greenstick*, when the bone is fractured half through on the convex side of the bend as in a green twig. Only seen in children. (4) *Comminuted*, where bone is broken into more than two pieces. (5) *Impacted*, where one fragment is driven into the other. (6) *Complicated*, where fracture is combined with injury to another important

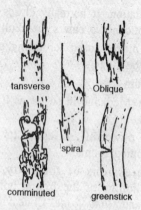

Types of fracture.

structure, *e.g.* artery, nerve, or organ. The type of break may be: (1) *Transverse*, due to direct violence applied at point of fracture. (2) *Oblique*, due to indirect violence, when a force applied at a distance causes the bone to break at its wekest part (3) *Spiral*, when a limb is violently rotated. (4) *Depressed fracture*, only of skull, when bone is driven inwards: it may be *guttershaped* with sharp depressed edge., or pondhaped with sloping edge; the latter is only in infants and due to birth injury.

Freudian. According to Freud's teaching. He taught that psychological disorders often resulted from unconscious sexual impressions during childhood. These he brought to consciousness through psychoanalysis. Dreams he said were the wish-fulfilment of repressed desires.

Friedman's test. Pregnancy test now obsolete. The urine of pregnant women contains an excess of secretion from the trophoblast, chorionic gonadotrophin, or APL principle. The urine is injected into an infantile rabbit. The rabbit is killed in 48 hours. If the woman is pregnant, characteristic changes will be seen in the overies of the rabbit.

Frustration. Disappointment experienced by a person who is thwarted and prevented by circumstances from achieving some desired object.

Fugue. A fleeing from reality as in hysteria. The patient has no recollection of his actions during this time.

Full time or term. The fetus is said to be at term when it is 20 to 21 in long, has both 'esticles descended (if a boy), and has finger-nails and toenails reaching to the ends of the digits. Such a child should weigh anything from 7 Ib upwards, and have been developing in the uterus for not less than forty weeks.

Fungi. A subdivision of Thallophyta including moulds, musrooms, rusts, yeasts, etc. Fungi are used as a source of protein and vitamins, certain enzymes, used in baking and brewing and antibiotics, notably penicillin. A few fungi cause disease in man.

Funnel chest. Also called pectus excavatum. A developmental deformity in which the sternum is depressed and the ribs and costal cartilages curve inwards.

Furuncle. A boil.

Furunculosis. The appearance of one or more boils.

Fusiform. Spindleshaped. Can describe a bacillus.

G

Gag. An instrument for keeping the mouth open.

Gaiactagogue. An agent that causes an increased flow of milk.

Galactocele. A cyst of the breast containing milk.

Galactorrhoea. Excessive flow of milk.

Galactosaemia. A metabolic disorder characterized by presence of galactose in the blood stream.

Gall. or *bile*. A secretion of the liver; it accumulates in the gall bladder.

Gall bladder. The membranous sac which holds the bile. *See Biliary ducts.*

Gallstone. Calculus in the gall bladder. If the stone passes into the cystic or common bile duct there is great pain, and if in the common bile duct, jaundice. *See colic.*

Galvanism. Therapeutic use of direct electric current, either continuous, or interrupted. Interrupted galvanism is used to stimulate denervated muscle.

Gamete. A sexual reproductive cell. *e.g.* sperm, ovum.

Ganglion. (1) A collection of nerve cells forming a nerve centre. They are found in the sympathetic nervous system and in other parts of the nervous system. (2) Surgically, a chronic synovial cyst generally connected with a tendon sheath; most common site, back of hand, near the wrist.

Ganglionectomy. Excision of a ganglion.

Gangrene. Massive necrosis of tissue as the result of reduced blood supply. *Dry g.* The arterial supply is increasingly diminished, the veins remaining patent. The part becomes dry and mummified. The comonest cause is senility. *Wet g.* is caused by a sudden interference with the arterial supply and the venous return, as may occur if a tourniquet is left on too long or in traumatic conditions. The part readily becomes infected. *Gas g.*, due to infection by a group of anaerobic gasforming organisms of which the bacillus Welchii is the best known. Wounds which have been in contact with soil are likely to be infected. The signs are a rise in the pulse rate after recovery from the initial shock, discolouration, oedema, discharge, and gas felt in the tissues. Anti-gas gangrene serum is given as a prophylactic and curative measure. Antibiotics are also prescribed.

Gargle. A liquid medicine for washing out the throat.

Gargoylism. Hurler's syndrome. A defect of skeletal development in which the skull is grossly deformed and the digital bones are bulbous, the hands assuming a claw-like appearance. There is often associated congenital heart disease, enlarged liver and spleen. and intellectual impairment.

Gasserian ganglion. A ganglion of the sensory root of the fifth cranial nerve deeply situated in the skull. It is sometimes operated on for the relief of intractable trigeminal neuralgia.

Gastrectomy. Removal of the stomach.

Gastric ulcer. ulceration of the mucosa lining the stomach.

Acute ulceration may be caused by ingested substances, *e.g.* aspirin. chronic ulceration may be due to reduced capacity of the epithelium to withstand the acid gastric secretion or to a tumour of the epithelium.

Gastrin. A hormone released by cells in the wall of the pyloric antrum. When it is distended. This stimulates the secretion of gastric juice by the secretory cels in the rest of the stomach.

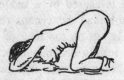

The genu-pectoral position

Gastritis. Inflammation of the epithelium lining the stomach.

Gaucher's disease. A very rare familian disease resulting in enlargement of the spleen with anaemia.

Gauze. Open mesh meterial used in surgical dressings.

Gavage. Forced feeding.

Geiger-Muller counter. Machine which detects and registers radio- activity.

Gigantism. Abnormal overgrowth of the body or of a limb, due to overactivity of the anterior lobe of the pituitary in young people. *See* ACROMEGALY.

Gigli's saw. An instrument for sawing through bone.

Gill, Liquid measure, $\frac{1}{4}$ pint.

Gingival. Relating to the gums.

Gingivitis. Inflammation of the gums.

Ginglymus. A hinge joint such as elbow or knee.

Girdle. Band encircling the body.

Glabella. Triangular space between the eyebrows.

Glairy. Slimy, albuminous.

Gland. A secreting organ. Some have ducts to carry away their secretion. e.g. the salivary glands. Others are ductless, *e.g.* the thyroid (*see* ENDOCRINE). Lymphatic glands manufacture leucocytes, filter the lymph and prevent the spread of infection.

Glanders. A febrile disease with inflammation of the nasal cavities, communicable to man from the horse, ass and mule. Often fatal.

Globulin. Group of proteins widely distributed in the body with numerous specialized functions. One group, the gamma-globulins are antibodies.

Globus hystericus. Hysterical choking feeling as if of a ball in the throat.

Glomerulonephritis. Acute inflammation of the kndney affecting all the glomeruli.

Glomerulus. The filtration unit of a nephron. It consists of a coil of fine capillaries lying in the invaginated blind end of the renal tubule.

Glossal. Relating to the tongue.

Glossectomy. Surgical removal of the tongue.

Glossitis. Inflammation of the tongue.

Glossodynia. Pain in the tongue sometimes associated with trigeminal neuralgia but often of unknown origin.

Glossopharyngeal. Relating to tongue and pharynx. *G. nerve* is the ninth cranial nerve.

Glossoplegia. Paralysis of the tongue.

Glottis. The aperture between the vocal cords in the larynx.

Glycerin. A sweet, colourless liquid, obtained from oils and fats and byproduct in the manufacture of soap. Used as an emollient in skin preparations.

Goblet cells. Pear-shaped cells in mucous membrane which secrete mucin.

Goitre. Enlargement of the thyroid gland. *Exophthalmic g.* Activity of the gland is increased, there is protrusion of the eyes, basal metabolic rate is high, increased pulse rate, tremor, sweating, nervousness, diarrhoea. *Parenchymatous g.*, uniform enlargement of the thyroid, very comon in young people. *Cystic g.*, may be (1) enlargement of a single vesicle, or (2) liquefaction of an adenoma. *Adenomatous g.*, encephaloid masses in gland substance which may be solid or cystic. *Malignant g.*, malignant growth of the thyroid.

Golgi's cells. Nerve cells with short processes found in the brain and spinal cord.

Gonadotrophins. Hormones which stimulate the gonads, e.g. FSH, LH.

Gonads. Reproductive glands: ovary of the female, testis of the male.

Gonococcus. The bacterium causing gonorrhoea. It is a Gram negative intra-cellular diplococcus.

Gonorrhoea. A venereal disease. An acute in Hammation, starting nearly always in the cervix or urethra, and due to the gonococcus. This disease is highly contagious. It may cause ophthalmia neonatorum. It may also cause ophthalmia in adults. By an ascending infection, in the female it may pass to the Falopian tubes and then cause peritonitis. The chief secondary complication of gonorrhoea is gonococcal arthritis, affecting mainly the large joints. The chief symptoms of gonorrhoea are profuse discharge and pain on passing water. Penicillin is administered.

Gout. Inherited defect of purine metabloism in which uric acid is in excess in the tissues. During acute attacks it is characterized by painful swelling of a joint, classically the big toe.

Graanfian follicles. Small bodies lying on the surface of the ovary, containing fluid and the egg cell. When the egg cell matures the follicle ruptures, setting it free to make its way to the fimbriated end of the Fallopian tube along which it travels.

Graefe's knife. Small knife used in operations for cataract.

Graft. Transplanted living tissue. *e.g.* skin, bone. *Skin g.* may be: (1) *Thiersch.* large pieces of epidermis with some dermis used chiefly for large areas. (2) *Wolfe.* the whole thickness of the skin is taken, used chiefly for small wounds. (3) *Pedicle,* used to reconstruct after burns or other severe injuries. The skin and underlying tissue is transplanted in stages. The graft retains its blood supply throughout. *Bone g.*, piece of bone removed, usually from the tibia, and secured to replace bone lost elsewhere.

Gram's stain. Bacteria which resist decolourization by alcohol after staining with methyl violet and Gram's solution are termed Gram positive, e.g. staphylococci, pneumococci. Those which are decolourized by alcohol are term Gram negative. e.g. B. coli, gonococci.

Gravitational ulcer. Ulcer of lower leg, often a complication of varicose veins.

Grey matter. Tissue of the CNS in which are situated numerous cell bodies of nerves, dendritic processes, glial cells, etc.

Grid radiotherapy. Irradiation through a sieve-like screen, *e.g.* lead, to improve tissue tolerance in palliative radiotherapy. Eczema of the hands, caused by frequent contact with flour and sugar.

Gutter splints. For limbs, made of wood, tin or some malleable metal, and grooved to fit the limb, and often lined with felt.

Gynaecology. The study and practice of the management and treatment of disorders affecting female organs, e.g. ovaries, uterus, vagina.

H

Haemangioma. Abnormal growth of blood vessels.

Haemarthrosis. Effusion of blood into a joint cavity.

Haematemesis. Vomiting blood from the stomach. The blood is dark. non-frothy, generally acid, and is mixed with traces of food. Common causes are ulcers or growths of the stomach.

Haematin. The iron containing pigment of haemoglobin.

Haematinic. A substance which increases the amount of haemoglobin in the blood, e.g. iron.

Haematocele. A tumour containing extravasated blood. *Pelvic h.*, a collection of blood in the pouch of Douglas, walled off by adhesions, usually caused by the leaking from a Fallopian tube, the seat of an ectopic gestation.

Haemochromatosis. Called also pigmentary cirrhosis or bronzed diabetes. The skin is pigmented due to the deposition of iron which is also present in the liver, heart and pancreas.

Haemodialysis. The removal of waste products such as urea and salt from the blood by circulating it through a dialyser for patients with renal failure.

Haemoglobin. The colouring matter of red blood cells, and the agent whereby oxygen is taken up from the air in the lungs and carried to the tissues. The amount of haemoglobin present in the blood can be estimated by a colour test, normal amount (14.6 grams per 100 ml) called 100 per cent haemoglobin.

Haemoglobinometer. An instrument for estimating the haemoglobin in the blood.

Haemolysin. Agent causing the breakdown of the red cell membrane.

Haemophilia. A congenital tendency to haemorrhage, the clotting power of the blood being deficient. It occurs only in males, but is transmitted through the females of the family.

Haemophiliac. A person suffering from haemophilia.

Haemophilus. Bacillus causing respiratory disorders such as the *H. influenzae*. H. pertussis is the cause of whooping cough.

Haemophthalmia. Haemorrhage into the eye.

Haemopoiesis. The process of formation of the blood cells, particularly the red blood cells. In the fetus, haemopoiesis occurs in the spleen and liver; in the adult, in the bone marrow.

Haemopoietin. A hormone produced by the action of the intrinsic factor in the gastric juice on the extrinsic factor, present in food. It is stored in the liver and activates the red bone marrow to manufacture red blood cells.

Haemoptysis. Coughing up of blood.

Haemorrhage. A flow of blood. It may be (1) *arterial*, occurring in spurts, and bright red in colour; (2) *venous*, occurring in a steady stream and dark in colour; (3) *capillary*, oozing from a large wound surface. Haemorrhage may be (1) *primary*, at time of injury; (2) *reaction-*

ary, within twentyfour hours of injury due to a rise in the blood pressure; (3) *secondary*, usually within seven to ten days of injury due to sepsis. Haemorrhage may be (1) *visible* or (2) *concealed*, into one of the cavities of the body and not appearing at the surface. The symptoms of concealed haemorrhage are pallor of skin and mucous membranes, quick, sighing respiration, rapid, small, weak pulse. restlessness, subnormal temperature, coldness, sweating and collapse. *See illustration* for pressure points for the arrest of haemorrhage, p. 160.

Haemorrhagic disease of newborn. Congenital abnormality of vitamin K metabolism which results in deficiency of prothrombin in the blood. As a result haemorrhages occur in the body following even slight trauma.

Haemorrhoidectomy. Surgical removal of haemorrhoids.

Haemorrhoids. Varicose rectal veins (piles).

Haemostasis. The prevention of haemorrhage or the measures taken for its arrest.

Haemostatic. An agent to arrest a flow of blood.

Hand. End of the arm. Its bones are the carpal, metacarpal and phalanges.

Handicapped. Mentally or physically disabled.

Hanot's disease. A rare type of cirrhosis of the liver of unknown origin.

Haploid. Having a set of unpaired chromosomes in the nucleus, characteristic of gametes.

Hare lip. A congenital slit in the upper lip, frequently associated with 'cleft palate'.

Harrison's sulcus. A groove extending from the level of the ensiform cartilage towards the axillae. It is produced in rickets.

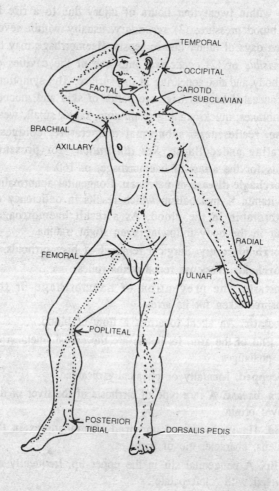

TEMPORAL

OCCIPITAL

FACIAL

CAROTID

SUBCLAVIAN

BRACHIAL

AXILLARY

RADIAL

FEMORAL

ULNAR

POPLITEAL

POSTERIOR
TIBIAL

DORSALIS PEDIS

*Arterial system. The arrows indicate points at which pressure
may be applied to check haemorrhage.*

Hartmann's solution. A saline solution containing sodium lactate. Used in acidosis.

Hashimoto's disease. A chronic thyroiditis due to autoimmunity to thyroglobulin. It causes myxoedema.

Hashish. An extract of Indian hemp, a drug included in the Misuse of Drugs Act. *See* CANNABIS INDICA.

Haustrations. Sacculations of the colon.

Haversian canals. The minute canals which permeate bone.

Hay fever. Allergic rhinitis caused by exposure of sensitized respiratory epithelium to certain dusts and pollens.

Head. That part of the body in which is the brain.

Headache. Pain in the head.

Health. A state of well-being with mind and body functioning at their optimum.

Heart. The muscular organ which pumps the blood through the system. The heart is situated behind the sternum, rather to the left, the apex of the heart being under the left breast. If the ear or a stethoscope be placed over a healthy heart, a dull thudding sound is heard, immediately followed by a short, sharper, crisper sound; a short pause follows and then the two sounds occur again. Each pair of sounds corresponds to one beat of the heart. *See* DIASTOLE and SYSTOLE. The heart consists of four chambers, the right and left atria and the right and left ventricles. The chambers are lined with the endocardium. Folds of endocardium form the valves of the heart. The heart is enclosed in a membranous sac, the pericardium.

Heart block. State of partial or complete prevention of the passage of the cardiac impulse through the atrioventricular, bundle. It is characterized by an extremely slow heart beat and pulse. *See also* ECG.

Heartburn. Burning sensation at lower end of the

oesophagus, due to acid regurgitation from the stomach.

Heart-lung machine. Machine used in cardiac surgery to oxygenate the blood.

Heat exhaustion. Condition caused by great heat when patient has rapid pulse, dysnoea and abdominal cramp due to excessive sweating and loss of sodium chloride.

Heatstroke. Hyperpyrexia due to failure of temperature regulating mechanisms of the body. Caused by extreme heat.

Helminthiasis. Infestation with worms.

Helminthology. The study of worms.

Hemeralopia, Partial blindness; patient can only see in broad daylight.

Hemi. Prefix meaning half.

Hemianopia. Loss of sight in half of the visual field.

Hemiatrophy. Atrophy of one side of the body only.

Heparin. An anti-coagulant derived from liver tissue. Given by intravenous or subcutaneous injection in doses based on laboratory determinations of patient's blood-clotting time.

Hermaphrodite. Abnormality of development in which an individual has tissue capable of producing both male and female gametes. It is associated with ambiguity of secondary sexual characteristics and the individual is generally sterile.

Hernia. Rupture. Protrusion of an organ from its normal position, most common in the case of the bowels. *Inguinal hernia* is through the inguinal canal. *Femoral* through the demoral ring. *Strangulated*, so tightly constricted that gangrene and acute intestinal obstruction results if operation does not relieve. *Scrotal* is hernia descending into the scrotum, and *umbilical* is hernia at the navel. A hernia not amenable to manipulation is termed irreducible. If the blood supply to this is interfered with it is termed strangulated. *Hernia cerebri* is protrusion of the brain through a wound in the skull. *Ventral h.*, of the ventral surface of the body such as an umbilical or incisional H., the latter is through an old scar.

Hernioplasty, Operation for hernia when the weak structures are repaired.

Heterogeneous vaccine. Made from some source other than the patient's own organisms; usually from a stock laboratory culture. Opposite to *autogenous.*

Hiccup, hiccough. Repeated spasmodic inspirtation associated with sudden closure of the glottis which gives rise to the characteristic 'hic' sound. It may be produced by irritation of the diaphragm but in most cases the cause is unknown.

Hidradenitis. A staphylococcal infection of the skin, occurring in the axillae.

Hidrosis. Sweating.

Higginson's syringe. The ordinary india-rubber syringe, consisting of two tubes, a bulb and valves to maintain flow in one direction only.

Hip. Upper part of thigh where it joins the pelvis.

Hip joint. Ball and socket joint between the head of the femur and the acetabulum. Congenital dislocation of h.j. Abnormality of development in which the head of the femur does not articulate with the acetabulum. The condition is almost always preventible if recognised within a few days of birth.

Hippocrates. A Greek physician who lived about 400 B.C. He is the father of modern medicine.

Hirschsprung's disease. Developmental abnormality in which there is a defect in the nerve supply to part of the terminal colon which causes an obstruction and results in dilation and hypertrophy of the more proximal segment (congenital megacolon).

Histamine. An organic base which is released from tissues, esp mast cells, following injury. It increases the permeability of blood cells and thus initiates the inflammatory reaction.

Hogben's test. A pregnancy test in which the patient's urine is injected into a toad. Now obsolete.

Homoeopathy. Medicine worked on the system of cures such as those started by Hahnemann homoeopathic medicines are mostly given in minute doses.

Homosexuality. A psychological abnormality in which sexual attraction is towards persons of the same sex.

Hormone. A substance produced in an endocrine organ which excites functional activity in another organ.

Horseshoe kidney. The most important of all serious forms of congenital abnormality of the kidney. The two kidneys are united at their lower poles and form a horseshoe mass generally at a lower level than normal. Possible cause of urinary infection.

Housemaid's knee. Inflammation of the bursa patellae, caused by constant kneeling on hard substances.

Houston's folds. Three oblique folds in the mucous membrane of the rectum.

Humanized milk. Cow's milk with reduced fat and increased sugar.

Humerus. The bone of the upper arm.

Humour. Any fluid of the body other than blood.

Hunger pain. A symptom of pepptic or duodenal ulcer. The pain is relieved on eating.

Hutchinson's teeth. A condition of the upper central permanent incisors: the cutting edge is smaller than the base, and therefore the teeth are peg-shaped. The edge is deeply notched a sign of congenital syphilis.

Hyalitis. Inflammation of the vitreous humour of the hyaloid membrane of the eye.

Hyaloid membrane, The glassy membrane which enclose the vitreous humour of the eye.

Hyaluronidase. An enzyme which, when injected subcutaneously, promotes absorption: in an injection 500 units aid absorption of 500 ml injection solution.

Hybrid. Offspring resulting from gametes which are genetically unlike.

Hydrocele. Swelling containing clear fluid. Most often applied to watery swelling of scrotum.

Hydrocephalus. A rare congenital disease seen in children. The sutures of the skull do not unite, the cerebrospinal fluid increases, causing the head to swell to an enormous size; often mental symptoms. *Acute h.* Distension of the ventricles, due to a cerebral tumour or meningitis.

Hydrocortisone. One of the adrenocortical hormones, similar in action to, but more powerful than, cortisone.

Hydrogen peroxide. H_2O_2. A valuable non-irritating and non- poisonous antiseptic. It effervesces in the presence of pus due to the liberation of oxygen. Usual strength 10 volumes, *i.e.* it contains ten times its volume of available oxygen.

Hydronephrosis. Distension of the pelvis and calyces of the kidney due to obstruction to the ureter. Prolonged back, pressure results in atrophy of the renal substance.

Hypermetropia. Long-sight, a visual affection. The opposite of myopia. Corrected by wearing a biconvex lens.

Hypermnesia. An exaggeration of memory involving minute details of a past experience. It may occur in mentally unstable individuals after a shock.

Hyperparathyroidis. Excessive secretion of the parathyroid glands.

Hyperphagia. Eating to excess.

Hyperphoria. Elevation of one visual axis above the other.

Hyperpiesis. Abonrmally high blood pressure.

Hyperpituitarism. Over-activity of the pituitary gland. Occurring in childhood the patient becomes a giant; in adult life, acromegaly develops.

Hyperplasia. Excessive growth of tissue.

Hyperpnoea. Respirations increased in rate and depth: a symptom of uraemia.

Hyperpyrexia. High fever, arbitrarily above 105° F. or 41° C.

Hypersecretion. Excessive secretion.

Hypersensitive. Abnormally sensitive *e.g.* to certain foodstuffs.

Hypertensin. Angiotensin.

Hypertension. Blood pressure above the normal limits, *i.e.* above 140/95 resting BP. Hypertension may be *primary* or *essential, i.e.* cause unknown, or *secondary* to artery obstruction, renal disease, endocrine disturbances and other factors.

Hyperthermia. Raised body temperature.

Hyperthymia. An overactive state of mind with a tendency to perform impulsive actions.

Hyperthyroidism, Excessive secretion of thyroid hormones.

Hypertonia. Excessive tonicity, as in a muscle or an artery.

Hypertrichosis. Excessive growth of hair, or growth of hair in unusual places.

Hypertrophy. Increase in size in response to demand on the structure, *cf.* hyperplasia.

Hypotensive drug. Term applied to drug which lowers the blood pressure.

Hypothalamus. A special area of grey matter in the floor of the third ventricle of the brain. Linked with the pituitary gland and also with the thalamus and the autonomic nervous system.

Hysterectomy. Removal of the womb by operation. Sub - total *hysterectomy* is removal of all the womb except the cervix. *Pan h.*, total hysterectomy. *Vaginal h.*, womb removed per vaginam.

Hysteria. A functional neurosis in which there is a reaction, never fully conscious on the part of the patient, to obtain relief from stress by the exhibition and experience of symptoms of illness.

Hysteroptosis. Uterine prolapse,

Hysterosalpingography. X-ray examination of the uterus, and the Fallopian tubes following the introduction of a contrast medium.

Hysterotomy. Incision into the uterus. The term usually excludes caesarean section.

Hysterotrachelorrhaphy. Repair of a lacerated cervix uteri.

Ichthyosis. Inherited defect of keratinization in which the skin is dry and scaly. The so-called acquired ichthyosis is similar in appearance but due to defective nutrition.

Icterus. Jaundice.

Icterus neonatorum. Jaundice of the new-born child. A slight degree of jaundice is not uncommon a few days after birth, and has no special significance; but serious and fatal cases also arise from umbilical sepsis, haemolytic disease of the newborn and other causes. *See* JAUNDICE.

Identical twins. Twins of the same sex and originating from the same ovum.

Ideo-motor. The association of movement with an idea. Psychologically it is rather like an obsession: an idea that leads to action against the will of the person.

Idiocy. Severe mental subnormality.

Idiopathic. Without apparent cause.

Idoisyncrasy. Individual character or property. Generally used in connection with unusual or unexpected response to drugs.

Ileectomy. Excision of the ileum.

Ileitis. Inflammation of the ileum. *Regional i.,* Crohn's disease. Characterized by localized regions of non-specific chronic inflammation of the terminal portion of the ileum. Occasionally other parts of the intestine are also affected. The cause is not known.

Ileocaecal valve. Valve at the junction of the large and small intestines.

Ileocolitis. Inflammation of the ileum and colon. A condition not uncommon in children.

Ileocolostomy. Surgical anastomosis between the ileum and the colon.

Ileoproctostmy. Operation when the ileum is joined to the rectum.

Ileorectal. Relating to the ileum and the rectum.

Ileosigmoidostomy. Implantation of the small intestine into the sigmoid flexure.

Ileostomy. Refers to an opening is made into the ileum for the discharge of intestinal contents, thereby bypassing the large bowel.

Ileum. The lower portion of the small intestine between the jejunum and caecum.

Ileus. Means obstruction of the bowel. Paralytic ileus caused by local inflammation affecting the nerve supply. It may be a complication of abdominal operations, particularly if the bowel has been extensively handled. It may be due to peritonitis.

Iliac crest. The highest portion of the ilium.

Ilium. The upper part of the innominate bone.

Illegitimacy. Born out of wedlock.

Illusion. Refers to a deceptive appearance. The misinterpretation of a sensory image.

Image. A mental picture of an external object.

Imbalance. Lack of balance.

Imbecility. Refers to a marked degree of mental incapacity.

Obsolete term.

Immune. Protected against a particular disease as by inoculation.

Immuinty. State of resistance to infection due to the presence of antibodies capable of combining with antigen(s) carried by the infecting organism and thus damaging the invader or neutralizing enzymes or toxins released by the organism. As well as viruses, bacteria and other parasites the body regards cells from a different individual, i.e. different genotype, as infecting organisms. Hence the difficulties of homo-grafting kidneys. In a wider, and less common usage of the term, immunity applies to all mechanisms, such as impermeability of the skin, antiseptic properties of sebum. disinfection of food by stomach acid, etc., which enable the body to resist infection.

Immunization. Refers to the process of increasing the state of immunity, either by contact with the infecting organism or some variant of it which is *Active i.* In *passive i.* there is receipt of an anti body. Active imunization is the priciple behind vaccination against smallpox, inoculation against diphtheria, tetanus etc. Passive immunization is temporary. The fetus is passively immunized by antibodies from the maternal blood enabling the new-born baby to resist infection for about six weeks after birth.

Immunology. The study of immunity.

Immunosuppression. Deliberate inhibition of normal ummune response, especially to permit successful organ grafting.

Impetrigo. A skin rash of an acute kind generally a streptococcal and staphylococcal infection. It is contagious.

Implantation. Refers to the act of setting in; grafting.

Implants. Pellets of drugs such as testosterone which are inserted under the skin from where they are slowly absorbed.

Impotence. Absence of power or desire for sexual intercourse.

Impregnation. The fertilization of an ovum by a spermatozoon. Permeation.

Implulse. A sudden driving force.

Inarticulate. (1) without joints. (2) Unable to speak clearly.

Incest. Sexual intercourse between near relatives.

Incisors. Chisel-shaped cutting teeth at the front of the mouth.

Inclusion bodies. Intracellular bodies found esp. in affected tissues in virus diseases.

Incubation. Hatching. Time between infection and the appearance of symptoms when it is assumed the infecting organisms multiply.

Incubator. Apparatus used to provide optimum conditions for incubation.

Incus. A small anvil-shaped bone of the middle ear.

Indian hemp. Cannabis indica. Also called marihuana.

Indicanuria. Excess of indican in the urine.

Indigestion. Failure of the digestive powers; dyspepsia.

Indol. A constituent of faeces formed by the putrefaction of protein. In cases of chronic constipation it is absorbed and excreted in urine as indican.

Indolent. Refers to a applied to a painless sore which is slow to heal.

Induction. In obstetrics, the artificial production of labour. In electricity, the production of currents in a closed circuit upon the appearance and disappearance of a magnetic or electric field in its neighbourhood.

Induration. The process of hardening; also, the state of being hardened, as in the early stage of inflammation.

Industrial disease. A disease due to a person's occupation such as silicosis found among silica workers, etc.

Inebriety. Habitual drunkenness.

Inevitable haemorrhage. Bleeding due to placenta praevia.

Infant. A newly born child: A term infant should be 50 to 53cm in length. In English law, a person under the age of legal maturity .*I. mortality. See* MORTALITY.

Infenticide. Murder of an infant.

Infantile eczema. Type of eczema affecting infants and children.

Infantile paralysis. Anterior polimoyelitis.

Infantilism. Persistence of shildish ways in an adult.

Infarct. A wedge-shaped area of dead tissue in an organ. The result of the clogging of an artery by an embolus or thrombus.

Infection. The communication of a disease from one patient to another. *Droplet i.* In the fine spray which is ejected from the mouth on talking, sneezing, coughing.

Infections disease. A communicable disease.

Infectious mononucleosis. Glandular fever. Probably a virus infection and characterized by malaise, pyrexia, muscle pains, sore throat enlargement of lymph glands and the spleen and an increase in the numbers of mononuclear white blood cells. Occasionally there is enlargement if the liver, jaundice and rash.

Inferior vena cava. The chief vein of the lower part of the trunk of the body.

Inferiority complex. Aggressive, extrovert behaviour compensating for feeling of inferiority.

Infertility. Inability to reproduce. It may affect either the male or the female.

Infestation. The invasion of the body by parasites such as lice.

Infiltration. (1) An effusion of fluid into the connective tissue. (2) Local spread of a malignant tumour.

Inflammation. The response of the tissues to an injury. The signs are heat, redness, swelling, pain, loss of function.

Influenza. Virus infection affecting the epithelium of the respiratory tract.

Infra-red. Electromagnetic waves with longer wave length than visible red light, *i.e.* photons with a lesser frequency than the lower end of the visible spectrum. Because it is easily absorbed infra-red radiation transfers heat to the absorbing materiala and is used therapeutically for this purpose.

Infundibulum. (1) a funnel-shaped orifice or passage. (2) Out- growth of floor of brain forming part of the pituitary gland.

Infusion. (1) Fluid allowed to flow into a vein (intravenous infusion) or under the skin (subcutaneous infusion) by the force of gravity. (2) Crude extract of material using boiling water *e.g.* tea is an infusion of tea leaves.

Ingestion. The taking in of food or other substances into the body.

Ingrowing toe-nail. Lateral extension of the nail bed.

Inhalation. Act of breathing in vapour or fumes by the mouth or nose a form of treatment frequently ordered in disorders of the throat or chest.

Inhaler. Apparatus for administering steam inhalation. The drug and boiling water are put into the container and the patient inhales through the mouthpiece.

Inherent. Inborn.

Injection, Introduced material under pressure into tissues.

Innervation. The supply of nerves or the conveyance of nervous impulses to or from a part. *Reciprocal i.* One set of muscles contracts whilst those opposing it relax.

Innocent. Not malignant.

Innominate artery. The large artery which arises from the arch of the aorta and divides into the right common carotid and right subclavian arteries.

Innominate bone. Bone forming anterior walls and sides of the pelvic cavity.

Inoculation. Introduction of microorganisms into tissue or culture media etc.

Inositol. Substance in vitamin B complex found in muscle and other animal tissue and also in seeds.

Inquest. A judicial inquiry into the cause of death.

Insanity. Madness. Severe mental disorder (an absolute term).

Insecticide. A preparation for destroying insects.

Insemination. Introduction of semen into the vagina. *Artificial i.* Injection of semen into vagina or uterus.

Insertion. The attachment of a muscle to the part it moves.

Insolation. Exposure to the sun's rays.

Insomnia. Sleeplessness; often a troublesome complication during convalescence.

Inspiration. Drawing air into the lungs.

Instep. Arch on the dorsal surface of the foot.

Instillation. Pouring in drop by drop. *e.g.* into eye.

Instinct. An inborn organization of perception, feeling and action, *e.g.* the sight of something which threatens life arouses the emotion of the fear and the instinct of flight.

Insuffliation. Blowing powder into a cavity of the body. The instrument used has a long tube or nozzle with a rubber bulb attached to the distal end.

Insula. Small part of the cerebral cortex lying deeply in the lateral sulcus.

Insulin. Secretion of the islets of Langerhans in the pancreas which exerts control over the metabolism of glucose in the body. Used as a subcutaneous injection for reduction of blood sugar in diabetes.

Insulinase. Enzyme which inactivates insulin.

Insulinoma. An adenoma of the islet cells of the pancreas.

Integument. The skin.

Intelligence. Certain mental ability involving resoning and recognition of pattern, etc., as distinct from memorization of information or other mental functions.

Intelligence quotient. The ratio of mental age to chronolological age.

Intelligence tests, Tests not based on a person's knowlege but on his ability to learn.

Intention tremor, Tremor which occurs only during active movement, symptomatic of Parkinsonism.

Intercourse, Communication. *Sexual i.* Coitus.

Intersex. Imperfect sexual differentiation of an individual into either male or female.

·Interstitial Keratitis. manifestation of syphilis consisting of inflammation of the cornea.

Intertrigo. Eczematous condition of deep crevices or folds of skin, due to retention of perspiration.

Intervertebral. Between the vertebrae.

Intestinal malabsorption. Malabsorption syndrome. Failure to absorb digested foodstuffs.

Intestinal obstruction. Obstruction to the passage of food or faeces through the intestine. Either due to physical block-age or absence of peristalsis.

Intestines. The alimentary canal from the doudenum to the anus.

Intima. Inner coat of arteries consisting of endothelium and its elastic fibre attachment to the connective tissue of the media.

Intoxication. Poisoning; drunkeness.

Intra-abdominal. Within the abdominal cavity.

Intramuscular. Within a muscle. Many injections are given intramuscularly but care must be taken with choice of site, because of danger of damaging nerves and blood vessels.

Introspection. State of mental self-examination.

Intumescence. Swelling, increase.

Intussusception. The reception of one part of the intestine (the intussusceptum) into another (the intussuscipiens); occurs most often between 3 and 9 months, and causing intestinal obstruction, with the passage of blood and mucus rectally and frequent vomiting. The treatment is immediate laparotomy.

Invagination. Turning inwards to form double-layered pouch.

Involuntary. Independent of the will *I. muscles* are innervated by the autonomic nervous system.

Involution. (1) A turning in. (2) The shrinking of the uterus and surrounding structures after labour. The uterus, from weighing 1 kg at labour, shrinks in six weeks to the weight of 50 g. Arrest of this process is called subinvolution.

Involutional melancholia. Depression due to hormonal

changes at the menopause. A similar syndrome occurs in males.

Iodine. A poisonous element obtained from the ashes of seaweed. A useful antiseptic for the skin.

Iodism. Iodine poisoning. Symptoms are those of a cold in the head with a pustular rash.

Ipsilateral. On the same side.

IQ. Abbreviation for intelligence quotient.

Iridectomy. Cutting off a pice of the edge of the iris to make an artificial pupil to the eye.

Iridocele. Protrustion of a portion of iris through a wound in the cornea.

Iridocyclitis. Inflammation of the iris and uveal tract.

Iridoplegia. Paralysis of the muscle which constricts or dilates the pupil.

Iris. The coloured circle surrounding the pupil of the eye. *See* EYE.

Iritis. Inflammation of the iris.

Irrigation. Washing out.

Irritant. Agent causing irritation, *i.e.* resulting in a response.

Ischaemia. Diminished supply of blood to a part.

Ischio-rectal abscess. A collection of pus in the fatty cavity on one or other side of the rectum. May burst externally through the skin or internally into rectum when a fistula-in-ano results.

Ischium. The lower and hind part of the innominate bone.

Ishihara test, Colour charts used to test for colour blindness.

Isotonic. Having the same osmotic pressure. Thus a solution which is isotonic with blood serum neither attracts fluid

from the vessels nor itself tends to pass through into
them.

Isotopes. Differing forms of the same element with different
atomic weights but the same chemical properties.
Radioactive i, Isotopes with radioactive properties, emit-
ting beta rays and sometimes gamma rays. Used to diagnose and treat disease.

Itching, Sensation, probably due to sub-threshold pain
stimuli, which is characterized by the *scratch* reaction.

IUD. INTRA-UTERINE.

Jacquemier's sign. Blueness of the vaginal walls seen in early pregnancy.

Jaundice. A syndrome which is characterized by increased levels of bile pigments in the blood and tissue fluids. These pigments are taken up by the tissues giving rise to a yellow colour of the sclera, skin and mucous membranes. The cause of jaundice may be obstructive, hepato-cellular or haemolytic (excessive destruction of red blood cells). Hepatocellular jaundice includes conditions such as infective hepatitis, a virus disease affecting the liver; toxic damage to the liver cells. *e.g.* acute yellow atrophy and other condition which reduce the efficiency of the liver in excreting bile pigments. Obstruction to any portion of the biliary tree may result in jaundice. The commonest cause of obstruction is gall stones.

Jejunum. That portion of the small intestine which lies between the duodenum and the ileum. *See* BOWEL.

jerk. A sudden contraction of muscle.

Jigger. A tropical sand flea (Dermatophilus penetrans) which is parasitic in man, burrowing into the toes. Another name is chigoe.

Joint. Point of contact of two or more bones. An articulation.

Jugular. Relating to the neck.

Jugular veins. Two large veins in the neck which convey most of the blood from the head.

Justo minor pelvis. From of CONTRACTED PELVIS.

K. Chemical symbol for potssium.

Kahn test. Refers a method of investigating the serum of patients suspected of sypto hilis. It is more convenient, simpler, and quicker than the wasserman Reaction, but should confirm rather than supplant it, the WR on the whole being more reliable.

Kala-azar. A tropical disease transmitted from man to man by sand-flies and is caused by the protozoon *leishmania donovani*. There is enlargement of the spleen, fever and anaemia.

Kaolin, China clay; a hydrated silicate of aluminium. It is an ingredient of cataplasma kaolini. *Heavy k.* is used to prepare k. poultice. *Light k.* is an adsorbent demulcent and is used in mixtures for diarrhoea.

Katathermometer. A wet and dry bulb thermometer for measuring the cooling and drying powers of the atmosphere, thus it is a test of the efficiency of the ventilation.

Kayser Fleischer rings. Brownish pigmented rings seen in the cornea of patients with wilson's disease.

Keller's operation. Operation to correct hallux valgus.

keloid. A connective tissue growth of the skin, arising always in a scar to some previous injury.

Kerateitasiu. Protrusion of the cornea.

Keratectomy. Surgical removal of part of the cornea.

Keratin. Fibrillar protein. It is produced by epithedial cells and is found in horns, hovves, hair and the protective covering of the skin.

Keratitis. Inflammation of the cornea.

Keratolytics. Agents such as salicylic acid which break down keratin.

Keratoma. A callosity or horny overgrowth.

Keratomalacia. Means softening of the cornea which may lead to ulceration and blindess. Occurs in association with vitamin A deficiency.

Keratome. Surgical knife used for incision of the cornea.

Keratometer. Ophthalmometer, which is used for measuring corneal astigmatism.

Keratoplasty. Corneal graft.

Keratosis. Skin disease with excess of horny tissue.

Kernicterus. Many areas of the brain, particularly the basal ganglia, central cerebellar nuclei, the medulla and hippocampus are stained yellow with bilirubin. The brain cells are damaged. A complication of haemolytic jaundice of the new born.

Kernig's sign. Refers to a sign of meningitis. It consists of an inability to extend the knee joint when the thigh is flexed to a right angle with the trunk.

Ketogenic diet. Diet loving high fat producing ketosis.

Ketonaemia. Ketone bodies in the blood.

Ketonuria. Ketone bodies in the urine.

Ketosis. Acidosis. The condition in which ketones are found in excess in the body.

Ketosteroids. Androgens secreted in the adrenals and testes, whose presence in the urine is an indication of the activity of these glands.

Kidneys. Two organs in the region of the hollow of the back which secrete the urine. *Artificial k.* Apparatus through which blood is pased and allowed to dialyse, across a membrane, usually a coiled tube, placed in a warm bath of saline. This process allows waste products and other materials to be removed from the blood and simulate the function of the kidneys.

Killian's operation. For suppuration in the frontal sinus. Removal of part of frontal bone to allow of complete drainage.

Kimmelstiel-wilson disease. Disease with glycosuria nephrotic symptoms proteinuria and oedema.

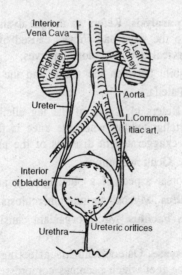

Anterior view of urinary tract

Kinaesthesis. Means the sense of muscular movement.

Kinase. Substances in the tissues which make proenzymes become enzymes.

Kirschner wire. Wire used in orthopaedic surgery to apply skeletal traction to a fractured bone.

Kiss of life. Mouth-to-mouth artificial respiration.

Klebs Loeffler bacillus. The bacillus of diphtheria. Also known as corynebacterium diphtheriae.

Klebsiella. Genus of abacteria which may cause respiratory infections.

Kleptomania. Obsessional neurosis manifested by compulsive stealing.

Klinefelter's syndrome. Chromosome abnormality causing infertility in the male due to congenital malformation of gonads.

Klumpke's paralysis, Refers to the paralysis of the flexor muscles to the wrist and fingers caused by injury to the eighth cervical and first dorsal nerves.

Knee, The joint between the femur and the tibia.

Knee cap. Patella.

Knee jerk. Refers to a jerk of the leg elicited by tapping on the patellar tendon when the knee is flexed. May be absent or exaggerated in diseases of the nervous system.

Knock-knee. Genu valgum.

Knuckle. Dorsal aspect of a phalangeal joint,

Koch's bacillus. Mycobacterium tuberculosis.

Koch-Weeks bacillus. Micro-organism causing acute conjunctivitis.

Köhler's disease. Osteochondritis affecting the scaphoid bone in the foot which becomes compressed and scleroti.

Occurs in children.

Koilonychia. The spoon shaped nails found in iron deficiency anaemia.

Koplok's spots. Small white spots to be found on the inner surface of the cheeks in measles, often before the skin rash appears.

Korsakow's syndrome. A confusional state especially as to recent events due to brain injury or toxic causes such as chronic alcoholism.

Kraurosis vulvae. Senile degeneration of the skin of the vulva.

Kretschmer's types. Classification of potential psychopathic ten dencies in relation to physical characteristics, *e.g.* pyknic type is short and fat with a tendency to manic depressive psychosis. Aesthetic type is tall and thin with a tendency to schizophrenia.

Krukenberg's tumour. Refers to a secondary carcinoma in the ovary, the primary usually occurring in the stomach.

Küntscher nail. Refers to an intramedullary nail used to fix fragments of fractured long bone in alignment.

Kupffer's cells. Star-shaped cells in the liver part of the reticuloendothelial system.

Kwashiorkor. Disease with wasting oedema, anaemia and enlargement of the liver due to lack of protein in the diet.

Kyphoscoliosis. Combined anteroposterior deformity (kyphosis) and lateral curvature (scoliosis) of the spine.

Kyphosis. Humpback, angular deformity of the spine. May be caused by Pott's disease.

Labia manora. Two large folds at the mouth of the pudendum; called also the *labia pudendi*.

Labia minora. Two smaller folds within the majora.

Labour. Refers to the progress of the birth of a child. There are three stages. (1) The dilatation of the cervix. (2) The passage of the fetus through the canal and its birth. (3) From the birth of the child to the expulsion of the placenta.

Labyrinth. The internal ear.

Labyrinthitis. Inflammation of the labyrinth of the ear causing vertgo.

Laceration. A lacerated wound with torn or irregular edges; not clean cut.

Lacrimal. Relating to tears and the glands which secrete them.

Lactalbumin. The albumun of milk. A protein.

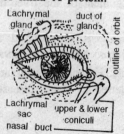

The lacrimal apparatus

Lactase. An enzyme of the succus entericus which converts lactose into glocose.

Lactation. The process or period of suckling.

Lacteals. The lymphatic vessels, which convey the chyle from the small intestine.

Lactic acid. An acid which is produced by the ermentation of lactose. The souring of milk is accompanied by the formation of this acid.

Lactiferous ducts. The canals of the mammary glands.

Lactobacillus. A non-pathogenic grampositive bacterium.

Lactogenic. Promoting the flow of milk. *L. hormone.* Prolactin. A hormone released from the anterior pituitary which causes milk production following parturition.

Lactose. A disaccharide sugar which is composed of glucose and galactose, which occurs in milk.

Laennec's cirrhosis. Refers to the commonest type of cirrhosis of liver commonly attributable to damage to the liver by high consumption of alcohol.

Lalling. Baby talk when the letter 'l' is used instead of the letter 'r'.

Lambliasis. Also called giardiasis. Parasitic infection of small intestine.

Laminectomy. Means excision of some of the vertebral laminae to gain access to the spinal cord or to relieve pressure on nerve roots as in prolapsed intervertebral disc.

Lancet. Refers to a sharp pointed two edged surgical knife.

Lancefield's groups. Classification of streptococci into groups of which Group A includes the common pathogenic haemolytic streptococcus.

Lancinating. Cutting or tearing, often applied to pain.

Lanette wax. A self-emulsifying wax which is used in water-micible ointment bases.

Langerhans's islets. Small areas of special cells in the pancreas, They secrete insulin.

Lanolin. Purified wool-fat. Used as the basis for various ointments.

Lansing virus. A strain of poliomyelitis virus.

Lanugo. The downy growth which covers an infant from the fourth month of gestation, but has mostly disappeared by term.

Laparotomy. Opening the abdominal cavity. Usually for investigation.

Lardaceous disease. Degeneration of the tissues till then resemble wax. Amyloid disease.

Laryngeal. Relating to the larynx. *L. stridor* Gasping respiration due to spasm of the glottis.

Laryngectomy. Removal of the larynx.

Laryngitis. Inflammation of the larynx, causing loss of voice, and in acute cases, with much oedema, threatening suffocation.

Larynology. Science of anatomy and diseases of the larynx.

Laryngopharynx. The lower part of the pharynx.

Laryngoscope. Instrument for examining a larynx.

Laryngostenosis. Stricture of the larynx.

Laryngo-tracheo-bronchitis. Acute viral inflammatory disease affecting the respiratory tract. Often occurs during influenza epidemic and affects principally young children.

Larynx. Refers to the part of the windpipe containing vocal cords. Voice sounds may be produced during expiration.

Laser. A very narrow and intense beam of light that will cut through metals.

Lassar's paste. Ointment containing zinc oxide, starch, salicylic acid, soft paraffin. Used for skin eruptions.

Lassitude. Feeling of weakness, a frequent feature of debilitating diseases wuch as anaemia.

Leather-bottle stomach. Refers to the loss of elasticity in the stomach wall resulting from infiltration by neoplastic cells.

Lecithin. A phospholipid.

Leech. Aquatic worm which is able to suck blood from the skin.

Leg. Anatomically the part of the lower limb from knee to ankle. *White l.* Condition caused by venous thrombosis in the lower limb. Sometimes seen after childbirth.

Legumin. A globulin which is derived from the seeds of various plants such as peas and beans.

Leishman-Donovan body. Eosinophilic bodies representing rounded forms of leishmania donovani found in the cells parasitized by kala-azar.

Leishmaniasis. Infection with organisms of the type which cause kala- azar and oriental sore.

Lembert's suture. Special suture used in stitching up the peritoneal coat of the intestine or other abdominal organs after any incision or injury.

Lennander's incision. Refers to an abdominal incision the right or left of the middle line down to the rectus; the inner edge of this muscle if then retracted and the posterior layer of its sheath incised as well as the peritoneum.

Lens. Transparent refractile tissue of the eye, which focuses the image on the retina.

Leon virus. A strain of poliomyelitis virus.

Leontiasis ossea. Refers to a disease in which the bones of the face are deformed and greatly increased in size; sometimes found in leprosy.

Leproma. Swelling in the skin found in certain cases of leprosy.

Leprosy. Refers to an infective disease, cutaneous in its earlier stages, but afterwards involving both soft tissus and bone. The first stage may last days or months; there are pains in the limbs, lassitude and feverish attacks. The second stage is eruptive and the blotches on the skin come and go. In the third stage the disease becomes either nodular (*lepra tuberculosa*) or blotched (*lepra maculosa*); if the blotches become white and anaesthesia sets in, it is called white leprosy. Leprosy, also called Hansens's lisease, was formerly treated with chaulmugra oil. Modern treatment is sulphone, therapy which can cure leprosy in its early stages.

Leptomeningitis. Inflammation of the pia mater and arachnoid coverings of the brain distinguished from pachymeningitis, in which the dura mater is the seat of inflammation.

Leptospira. Type of spirochaete. Notably *L. lcterohaemorrhagicae* which causes Weil's disease.

Leriche syndrome. Obstruction to the flow of blood at the lower end of the aorta giving rise to intermittent claudication.

Leasbianism. A female homosexual relationship.

Lesion. Refers to any injury or morbid change in the function or structure of an organ.

Lethal. Deadly, fatal.

Lethargy. Drowsiness.

Leucin. An amino-acid.

Leucocyte. A white blood cell.

Leucocythaemia. Morbid increase of the white cells of the blood. Same as leukaemia.

Leucocytolysis, Destruction of leucocytes.

Leucocytosis. An increase of white cells of the blood; usually occurs in sepsis and is then a defensive mechanism.

Leucoderma, Refers to the condition in which there are patches of skin which are defectively pigmented and consequently pale in colour.

Leuco-erythroblastic anaemia. Descriptive term applied to the appearance of nucleated red cells and primitive white cells in the circulation. It is due to neoplastic infiltration of bone marrow.

Leuconychia. Curved white lines on the finger-nails showing inter- rupted nutrition.

Leucopenia. Diminution of the number of white cells in the blood.

Leucopoiesis. Refers to the formation of white blood cells.

Leucorrhea. A whitish mucoid discharge from the vagina.

Leucotomy. Transection of nerve fibres passing to and from a lobe of the brain. Usually *prefrontal leucotomy*, an operation undertaken to relieve certain types of mental disorder in which the prefrontal lobes are surgically isolated from the rest of the brain.

Leukaemia. A disease of blood forming organs, characterized by increase of white cells of the blood. *Lymphatic l.* That in which large number of primitive lymphocytes appear in the blood. *Myeloid l.* That in which primitive polynorphonuclear leucocytes appear in large numbers. *Monocytic l., Eosinophilic l.,* as for the other forms, but exhibiting monocytes and eosinophils respectively.

Leukoplakia. A smooth glazed white state of the tongue which may precede cancer of that organ. A similar condition of the vulva is also found in women.

Levator. Refers to a muscle which lifts up a part. *Levator ani:* muscle of the pelvis which plays an important part in keeping pelvic viscera in position. *Levator palpebrae* superioris: muscle which raises the upper eyelid.

Levulose. Fruit sugar or fructose. *L. tolerance test.* In the normal individual there is little or no rise in the blood sugar taken 1 hour after 100 grams of levulose. In hepatic insufficiency the blood sugar will show an increase of 30mg per 100ml in the first half-hour and may later rise much higher.

Lice. Plural of louse.

Lichen. A term for skin diseases of which the striking feature is chronic inflammatory papules. Lichen planus: showing papules, which are angular. lilac in colour, often with a depression in their centre and in some lights shiny. Usually affects flexor aspects of forearms, back of neck, and inner side of thighs.

Lie of fetüs. The position of the fetus in the uterus is termed its lie, i.e. transverse lie, vertical lie.

Lieberkuhn's glands. Tubular glands of the small intestine which secrete the intestinal juice.

Ligament. A tough band of fibrous tissue connecting together the bones at the joints.

Ligation. The application of a ligature.

Ligatures. Threads of silk, wire, catgut, fascia, nylon, etc., used to tie arteries stitch tissue, etc.

Light adaptation. The adaptation of the pupil of the eye to light incident on the retina. Also termed light reflex.

Lightening. Relief of pressure in upper part of abdomen during last few weeks of pregnancy when fetal head enters the pelvis.

Lightning pains. Shooting, cutting pains felt in some cases of tabes dorsalis.

Lime. Calcium oxide. Lime salts increase the coagulability of the blood; they take part in the formation of bone, and are a component part of many toinc medicines.

Lime water. A solution of calcium hydroxide in distilled water. Used as a diluent for milk, and generally to counteract acidity.

Linctus. A syrup, usually applied to a cough mixture to be taken in small doses.

Linea nigra. A pigmented line seen in pregnant women running in midline from above the umbilicus to the symphysis pubis.

Liniment. A liquid preparation for application to the skin with friction.

Linolenic acid. A constituent of vegetable fats, essential for health.

Linseed. Seeds of the flax plant.

Lint. Loosely woven cotton material, having one side smooth and the other rough. The smooth side is applied next to the skin.Used for surgical fomentations and kaolin poultices.

Lipaemia. Presence of excess of fat in the blood.

Lipase. An enzyme in the pancreatic secretion which splits fat into glycerin and a fatty acid. *Syn* steapsin.

Lipo atrophy. Loss of subcutaneous fat. A complication which may arise in sites of insulin injections.

Lipodystrophy. Refers to a disorder of fat metabolism which most commonly affects women who show little fat above the waist but are obese around the buttocks and legs.

Lipoidosis. Disturbance in metabolism of lipoids.

Lipoids. Substances (*e.g* . lecithin) which resemble fats, in being dissolved by organic solvents such as alcohol and ether. They occur in living cells.

Lipoma, Tumour of fat cells.

Lipotrophic subastances. Factors such as choline and methionine, found in the diet and preventing excess of fat being deposited in the liver.

Liquor amnii. The watery fluid by which the fetus is surrounded.

Liquor folliculi. Fluid in a graafian follicele.

Liquores. Solutions of active substances in water Liquor calcis saccharatus lime-water.

Listerism. The principles of antisepic surgery.

Liston's splint. To immobilize the hip; made of wood. Little used now.

Lithagogues. Drugs which expel or dissolve stones.

Lithiasis. Formation of stone.

Litholapaxy. Operation for crushing a stone in the bladder and removing the fragments at the same time.

Lithopaedion. A calcified fetus in the abdominal cavity.

Lithotomy. Operation of cutting into a bladder to remove a stone.

Lithotomy position. Patient supine with Thighs and knees flexed. The hips must be abducted.

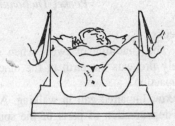

lithotomy position

Lithotrite. An instrument for crushing stones in the bladder. It is passed through the urethra.

Lithotrity. operation of crushing a stone in the bladder.

Lithuria. Passing gravel or crystals of uric acid with the urine.

Litmus. A blue pigment turned red by acids. L. paper. Paper impregnated with litmus; used fot testing urine and gastric secretion. A red litmus paper is turned blue by an alkali.

Little's disease. Spastic paraplegia or diplegia of infants due to birth injury or faulty development of the brain.

Litter's hernia. A diverticular hernia.

Liver. Large organ occupying the upper right portion of the abdomen. It has many important functions including the secretion of bile, the manufacture of serum albumin and the storage of glycogen, etc.

Loa loa. One of the parasites causing filariasis.

Lobar. Pertaining to a lobe.

Lobe. Rounded division of an organ.

Lobectomy. Excision of a lobe.

Lobule. Small lobe.

Localized. Limited to a certain area; not widespread.

Lochia. The vaginal discharge following delivery. For the first day or two is almost pure blood, but in normal cases becomes rapidly brown and then paler and ceases in a few weeks.

Locked twins. The condition of twins when some part of one absolutely prevents the birth of the other by causing complete impaction.

Locomotor ataxia. Impaired gait in walking. A chronic disease due to degeneration of parts of the spinal cord and nerves.

Loculated. Divided into many cavities.

Locum tenens. A practitioner who temporarily takes the place of another.

Loin. The lateral portion of the back between the thorax and pelvis.

Longevity. Long life.

Long sight. Hpermetropia.

Lordosis. Undue curvature of the spine with the convexity forwards; an exaggeration of the normal curve of the lumbar part of the spine.

Loreta's operation. Forcible dilatation of the pylorus for stricture.

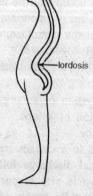

Lardosis

Lotion. A medicinal solution for external use.

Loupe. Magnifying lens used in ophthalmology.

Lovset's manoeuver. An obstetrical manoeuver used to deliver breech presentations with extended arms.

Lower motor neurone disease. Disease affecting the lower motor neurone libres. they arise from cell bodies in the anterior horns of the spinal cord and pass to the motor end plates of the muscles which they innervate. Lesions of the lower motor neurones result in paralysis and wasting of the muscles.

Lower uterine segment. Refers to that portion of the uterus, consisting of the cervix and the lower end of the body, which undergoes dilatation during labour.

LSD. Lysergic acid. One of the hallucinogenic group of drugs.

'Lubb-dupp. The heart sounds. The first is heard when the atrio- ventricular valves close the second on closure of the semilunar valves.

Ludwig's angina. An acute inflammatory condition in the sublingual and submaxillary regions.

Lumbago. Refers to the painful condition of the lumbar muscles, due to inflmmation of their fibrous sheaths. May be caused by a displaced intervertebral disc.

Lumbar. Pertaining to the region of the loins.

Lumbar puncture. The operation of tapping the cerebrospinal fluid in the lumbar region.

Lumbar sympathectomy. Operation to remove the sympathetic chain in the lumbar region.

Lumen. The cavity inside a tube.

Lungs. The two organs of respiration, situated in the right and left sides of the cavity of the chest.

Lunula. White crescent at the root of the nail.

Lupus erythematosus. A disorder classed with the so-called collagen diseases. A localized form may affect the skin of exposed regions. The generalized form is known as systemic lupus erythe matosus. The clinical manifestations of the disease are very varied. The criterion of diagnosis is the presence of LE cells in peripheral blood. LE cells are white cells which have ingested nuclear material.

Lupus vulgaris. Tuberculosis affecting the skin.

Luteinizing hormone. Hormone of the anterior pituitary gland stimulating the formation of corpus luteum in the ovary.

Luteotrophin. Pituitary hormone responsible for subsequent growth and development of corpus luteum, after its formstion by the follicle-stimulating hormone and the luteimzing hormone.

Luxation. Dislocation of joint.

Lymph. That part of the blood plasma which has passed through the walls of the capillaries, bathing the tissue cells, giving them nourishment and taking away waste products. It is also found in the lymphatic vessels and serous cavities.

Lymphadenitis. Inflammation of the lymphatic glands.

Lymphadenoma. Also called Hodgkinym's disease. Serious disease characterized by enlargement of the lymphatic glands and progressive anaemia usually with enlargement of the spleen. There are often remissions, and it can be checked for a time by chemotherapy, x-rays, and surgical removal of localized groups of glands.

Lymphangiectasis. Dilated state of lymphatic vessels.

Lymphangioma. Tumour composed of lymphatic vessels.

Lymphangioplasty. An operation for the relief of lymphatic obstruction.

Lymphangitis. Inflammation of lymphatic vessels.

Lymphatics. Small vessels pervading the body and containing lymph.

Lymphocytes, One of the normal varieties of white blood cells. Lymphocytosis, excess of these cells in the blood; found in leukaemia, whooping cough, tuberculosis and lymphadenoma. *Lymphopenia* deficiency of lymphocytes.

Lymphocythaemia. Increase of lymphocytes in to bloodstream.

Lymphocytosis. Lymphocythaemia.

Lymphogram. Refers to the method of demonstrating the lymphatic system following the injection of contrast medium opaque to x- rays.

Lymphogranuloma inguinale. A venereal disease found esp. In the tropics.

Lymphoid. Having the character of lymph.

Lymphoma. Tymour of lymphatic tissue.

Lymphosarcoma. A sarcoma originating in lymphatic tissue.

Lysergic acid. See LSD.

Lysins. Antibodies which are able to dissolve cells. *Haemolysins,* those able to dissolve red blood cells. *Bacteriolysins,* those able to dissolve bacteria.

Lysis. Dissolution. Decline of a fever.

Lysozyme. Bactericide found in tears, nasal mucus and other secretions.

M

McBurney's point. On line from umbilicus to anterior superior iliac spine, at outer edge of rectus muscle; corresponds to base of the appendix, and pressure here will give rise to pain when appendix is inflamed.

Mackenrodt's ligaments. Also called transverse cervical or cardinal ligaments. One of the chief supports of the uterus.

Macrocytes. Abnormally large red cells present in the blood in certain types of anaemia, including pernicious anaemia.

Macroglossia. Hypertrophy of the tongue.

Macroscopic. Visible to the naked eye.

Macula. A spot discolouring the skin. *M. lutea*, central spot of the posterior surface of the retina, just lateral to the optic disc marked by a small depression, and where vision is most acute.

Mal. Sickness. Mal de mer, sea sickness. Grand mal major epilepsy.

Malaria. A disease due to a parasite introduced into the blood by certain mosquitose.

Malignant. Virulent, fatal. A *malignant tumour* or growth is one which if not totally removed will spread locally and also cause similar growths in other part of the body until the patient dies, *e.g.* carcinoma, sarcoma.

Malignant hypertension. Hypertension associated with papilloedema and renal failure.

Malignant pustule. Anthrax contracted from cattle,causing gangrenous carbuncle.

Malnutrition. A state of undernourishment or imperfect nutrition.

Malocclusion. Bad contact between the masticating surfaces of the upper and lower teeth.

Malpighian corpuscle. Mesh of capillaries which act as a filtering coil for blood passing through the kidneys.

Malpresentation. Any presentation other than the vertex, of the fetus at the onset of labour.

Malt. Grain of barley which has begun to sprout and has then been dried. It contains a ferment (malt diastase) which converts starch into sugar.

Maltase. An enzyme of the succus entericus which converts maltose into glucose.

Maltose. A disac-charide composed of two molecules of glucose.

Mamilla. The nipple.

Mammae. the breasts, or milk-supplying glands.

Mammaplasty. Plastic surgery on the breasts.

Mammary. Relating to the breasts.

Mammography. To demonstrate tissue changes in the breast— xeroradiography frequently used for this technique.

Manchester repair. A type of gynaecological operation for uterovaginal prolpase.

Mania. Pathological combination of elation and energy. The patient is uncontrollably excited.

Manic depressive psychosis. A mental illness when intense excitement alternates with depression.

Mantoux test. Test of the body's reaction to anti-genic material prepared from PPD. This material called tuberculin is injected intradermally in serial dilutions (1.0 TU; 10.0 TU; 100 TU in 0.1 ml isotonic saline). A localized inflammatory reaction within 48 hours signigies a positive response. *Heaf test.* A similar test for the same purpose. Tuberculin is injected by special 'gun'.

Marble bone disease. Disease which may be familial, with osteosclerosis of the entire skeleton, the spongy part of the bone becoming compact. There is also anaemia.

Marrow. The soft substance which fills the medullary canal of a long bone and the small spaces in cancellous bone. The red cells of the blood are formed in the red bone marrow. Yellow marrow conatains fat.

Marrow puncture. investigative procedure involving the aspiration of marrow cells, usually by puncturing the sternum with a needle.

Masochism. A delight in being tortured or humiliated from which a sexual pleasure may be derived.

Mason's gag. A mouth gag.

Massage. Manipulation and rubbing of body designed to promote blood flow.

Masseter. A strong facial muscle which moves the lower jaw.

Mastalgia. Pain in the breast.

Mast-cells. Cells containing heparin and histamine, lining the walls of small blood vessels.

Mastectomy. Surgical removal of the breast. *Radical m.* The breast is removed together with the lymph glands of the axilla and the pectroal muscle.

Mastitis. Inflammation of the breast.

Mastodyina. Pain in the breasts often in the premenstrual phase.

Mastoid. Literally, breastlike. The *mastoid process* is the projecting portion of the temporal bone behind the ear; it contains numerous air spaces including the mastoid antrum.

Masturbation. Excitation of one's own genitals to produce an orgasm.

Materia medica. Branch of medical study dealing with the nature and use of drugs, i.e pharmacology and therapeutics.

Matress suture. A continuous stitch through both the skin edges.

Maxilla. The upper Jaw bone.

Measles, morbilli. An infectious disease common in children. Incubation period 10 to 12 days. Early symptoms are those of a cold, sore throat, cough and rise in temperature, Koplik's spots. The rash appears on the fourth day, about the neck and behind the ears, gradually spreading to the rest of the body and extremities. The normal is reached about the seventh or ninth day. Most infectious period is before the rash appears. *German measles*, Rubella.

Meckel's diverticulum. A small blind protrusion occasionally found in the lower portion of the ileum. In rare cases it produces acute intestinal obstruction by strangulating an adjacent coil of gut.

Meconium. A black, sticky substance voided from the bowels of an infant during the first day or two after its birth.

Mediastinum. The space in the chest between the two lungs. It contains the heart glands and great vessels.

Medical jurisprudence. Medicine as it is connected with the law; for instance, in case of suicide or murder.

Medicament. Any medicinal drug or application.

Medicated. Impregnated with a medicament.

Medication. Giving a medicine to a patient. Pre-operative m. One given before an operation as a basal anaesthetic.

Medicinal. Pertaining to the science of medicine or to a drug.

Medicine. the treatment of disease. A drug used to prevent or treat disease. Term often used for diseases for which surgery is not required.

Medico-chirurgical. Relating to both medicine and surgery.

Medico-social worker. Specially trained worker in hospital concerned with the patient in the community. Formerly called hospital almoner, now known as a hospital social worker.

Medulla. Latin for marrow. Term also applied to central part of various organs e.g. Kidney, adrenal gland.

Medulla oblongata. The lowest part of the brain where it passes through the oframen magnum and becomes the spinal cord. It contains the vital ventres which govern circulation and respiration.

Medullary. Relating to the marrow.

medulloblastoma. Malignant tumour, from embryonic cells of neuro- epithelial origin, occurring in the cerebellum.

Megalomania. Mental condition with delusional ideas of personal greatness.

Meibomian glands. Sebaceous glands of the eyelids, M. cyst chalazion.

Meigs's sydrome. Ascites and hydrothorax associated with ovarian fibroma.

Melaena. Black tarlike stools, due to the presence of blood which has undergone changes in the alimentary tract. The blood is often from a gastric or duodenal ulcer.

Melancholia. Morbid depression, a form of mental illness. There is ofter a strong suicidal tende4ncy.

Melanin. A name for the dark pigments found in the eye, skin, hair; pigmentation may be markedly increased in Addison's disease.

Melanoma. A tumour containing black pigment, melanin. May start as innocent pigmented wart, but possesses tendency to malignancy. (Malignant melanoma or melanotic carcinoma).

Meniere's disease. Giddiness resulting from disease of the internal ear or the equilibrating mechanism of the brain.

Meaninges. The membranes surrounding and covering the brain and spitail cord. They are, from without: the dura mater the arachnoid, the pia mater.

Meningioma. Tumour derived from the meninges.

Meningism. Syndrome characterized by symptoms and signs of meningitis but occurring in the absence of any causative organism. Probably a non-specific inflammatory reaction of the meninges to circulating toxins or some other trauma.

Meningitis. Inflammation of the meninges due to infection by organisms. Acute bacterial or viral meningitis is characterized by fever, headache, vomiting, backache and development of a stiff neck. Stupor, coma, convulsions may follow. A more insidious onset is sometimes seen in tuberculous meningitis.

Meningocele. Protrusion of meninges from a bony defect

usually in the spine, *e.g.* Spina bifida.

Meningococcus. A micro-organism the cause of cerebrospinal fever.

Menopause. Cessation of menstruation. Ovulation stops and reproductive life ends. It usually occurs between 40 and 50 years of age and is associated with alterations in hormonal balance which sometimes produce troublesome symptoms such as hot flushes, etc.

Menorrhagia. Exessive menstrual bleeding.

Menses. The menstrual flow.

Menstruation. Monthly discharge of uterine mucosa iwth resultant bleeding which occurs in the absence of pregancy in sexually mature women.

Mercurialism. Chronic poisoning by mercury. Occurs in workmen who labour with the metal, or inhale its vapours. *Symptioms:* (1) soreness of gums and loosening of teeth; (2) increased salivation; (3) foetor of breath; (4) griping and diarrhoea.

Mesosalpinx. The part of the broad ligament which lies immediately below the Fallopian tubes.

Mesovarium, A short perirtoneal fold connecting the ovary to the posterior layer of the broad ligament.

Metabolism. The biochemical processes taking place in the tissues of a living organism. Building up processes known as anabolism. Breaking down processes known as katabolism.

Metacarpals. The five bones of the hand joining the fingers to the wrist.

Metamorphosis. Transformation.

Metaphysis. Part between the shaft, disphysis, and the end, epiphysis, of the long bones.

Metaplasia. Conversion of one tissue into another.

Metastasis. Transfer or spreading of a disease from one organ to another which is remote. A malignant growth is spread in this way.

Metatarsalgia. Pain in the fore part of the foot.

Metatarsals. The five bones of the foot between the tarsus and the toes.

Meteorism. Distension of the intestines by gas.

Methaemoglobin. Altered haemoglobin producing cynosis.

Methaemoglobinuria. The presence of methaemoglobin in the urine.

Methandienone. An anabolic steroid derived from testosterone.

Methionine. An essential amino-acid containing sulphur. Used in liver damage and hepatitis.

Methylated spirit. Ordinary ethyl alcohol to which some methyl alcohol has been added in order to give it a nauseous taste and odour.

Metritis. Inflammation of the womb.

Metrocolpocele. Protrusion of the uterus into the vagina, the wall of the vagina being pushed in advance.

Metropathia, haemorrhagica. Excessive menstrual bleeding due to excess of oestrin and associated with follicular ovarian cysts.

Metrorrhagia. Bleeding from the uterus, other than at the menstrual period. It should always be investigated, as it is usually due to some pathological condition.

Michel's clips. Small metal clips used for suturing skin wounds after surgical operations. A special forceps is necessary for their removal.

Microcytic anaemia. Due to iron deficiency. The red cells in the blood are smaller than normal. The treatment is to give large doses of iron.

Micro-organism. Any microsopic plant or animal.

Microphthalmos. Abnormal smallness of eyes.

Microsporon. A fungus causing disease of the skin and hair.

Microtome. An instrument for cutting fine sections for microsopic examination.

Micturition. The act of passing urine.

Midbrain. Part of the brain between the forebrain and hindbrain.

Midriff. The diaphragm.

Midwife, A woman who conducts the confinement of another.

Midwifery, The art and science of the conduct of pregnancy, labour and the puerperium.

Migraine, Paroxysmal attacks of headache, usually with nausea and often preceded by disorders of vision. Migraine is usually unilateral.

Miliaria papillosa, Prickly heat; an affection due to a disorder of the sweat glands. Their ducts are obstructed.

Milk, The secretion of the mammary glands. The average composition is:

	Human Milk %	Cow's Milk %
Protein:		
Lactalbumin	1.4 ⎫ 2	.75 ⎫ 4
Casein	.6 ⎭	3.25 ⎭
Fat	4	4
Carbohydrate	6	4
Salt	.2	.7
Water	87.8	87.3

Human milk is neutral or slightly alkaline. Cow's milk is usually slightly acid by the time it reaches the consumer. Specific gravity 1026 to 1036.

Milk sugar. The first set of teeth.

Millin's prostatectomy. In this operation the bladder is not incised but the prostate gland is enucleated from around the neck of the bladder. Also called retropubic prostatectomy.

Milton. Proprietary antiseptic containing sodium hypochlorite.

Mitral valve. The valve of the heart between the left atrium and the left ventricle. Disease of this valve may give rise to *mitral stenosis* when there is narrowing of the orifice of the valve or mitral *regurgitation* or *incompetence* when the valve fails to close properly.

Mittelschmerz. Pain occurring at the time of ovulation allegedly due to peritoneal irritation by blood from the ruptured follicle.

Molar teeth. The grinders.

Mole. Pigmented raised area of skin, which may also be hairy. (2) In obstetric practice, a tumour composed of coagulated blood, fetal membranes and the embryo; due to haemorrhage into a gestation sac, and followed sooner or later by abortion.

Molluscum. Skin disease, either *contagiosum,* common in childhood, or *fibrosum,* involving the formation of overgrowths of fibro-cellular tissue.

Monckeberg's arteriosclerosis. Sclerosis of the medium and small arteries with extensive degeneration of the middle muscle lining, with atrophy and calcareous deposits in the muscle cells.

Mongolism, Down's syndrome. Due to abnormality of chromosome 21 occurring during meiosis. A chromosome pair fails to separate with the result that the child has a chromosome too may. *i.e.* 47 instead of 46. Mongols usually have slanting eyes, short head, hypotonia and a low IQ.

Mono-amine oxidase inhibitor. Drug which relives depression by preventing breakdown of serotonin and other amines in brain tissue, *e.g.* phenelzine. During treatment, alcohol and foods rich in tyramine, *e.g.* cheese, should be avoided.

Monster. An abnormal individual owing to fetal maldevelopment.

Mons veneris. The eminence over the os pubis in women.

Montgomery's glands. Small prominences about the nipple, which become more evident during preganncy and lactation.

Mooren's ulcer. Basal cell carcinoma affecting the cornea.

Morbid. Diseased, disordered, pathological.

Morbilli. Measles.

Morphine. An alkaloid obtained from opium, used as a sedative or anodyne.

Morphinism. Chronic poisoning from indulgence in the drug.

Morphoea. Scleroderma affecting the skin only. Patches of atrophic, depigmented skin overlie connective tissue which has lost its elasticity.

Mortality. Death rate. The annual death rate in this country is the no. of registered deaths × 1,000 divided by the mid-year population. The Infant M. Rate is the no. of deaths of infants under 1 year × 1,0000 divided by the no. of registered live births. The *Maternal M. Rate* is the no. of deaths of women ascribed to pregnancy or childbearing × 1,000 divided by the no. of registered live and stillbirths.

Mortuary. A place where dead bodies are kept.

Motor nerves. Those nerves which, passing *from* a nerve centre, effect a response in the motor organ (a muscle or a gland); the opposite to sensory nerves, which, passing to a nerve centre. convey a sensation.

Motor neurone disease. The disease of unknown cause characterized by degeneration of the anterior horn cells of the spinal cord, the motor nuclei of the cranial nerves and the corticospinal tracts; also called progressive muscular atrophy and amyotrophic lateral sclerosis.

Mould. Any minute fungus.

Moulding. The alteration in shape of the infant's head produced by the pressure it is subjected to whilst being driven through the birth canal.

Mountain sickness. Vomiting, tachycarda, breathlessness.

Mucilage. Aqueous solutions of gum or starch.

Mucin. An albuminoid constituent of mucus.

Mucous membrane, A surface which secretes mucus. The lining of the alimentary canal, air passages, and urinogenital organs: merges into true skin at the various onfices of these canals. *Mucous polypus*, a small outgrowth from the mucous surface of the cervix uteri or of the nose.

Mucus. A viscid fluid of the body secreted by the mucous membranes. Mucus in the urine shows as a transparent, cloudy sediment, easily dispersed by shaking the vessel.

Multiple myeloma. Neoplasm of plasma cells which infiltrate and replace the bone marrow. Characteristic features and anaemia, bone pain, and large quantities of circulating globulins of an abnormal type which may be excreted in the urine.

Multiple pregnancy. Twins, triplets, or any larger number of fetuses gestated together by one mother.

Mumps. Infectious parotitis, inflammation of the parotid glands. Long incubation period, twelve to twenty-eight days, and quarantine must therefore be most carefully enforced. A complication not uncommon is acute swelling of the testes with great pain; and occasionally acute ovaritis in females.

Murmur. Abnormal sound of the heart or the lungs heard upon auscultation.

Muscarine. A poisonous alkaloid which is a product of putrefaction and is occasionally found in mushrooms.

Muscle. Specialized tissue composed of highly contractile cells. There are three varieties of muscle in the body: (1) Striated, voluntary muscle. (2) Smooth, involuntary, and (3) Cardial muscle. *M. atrophy peroneal.* Charocot-Marie-Tooth disease. An inherited condition in which there is degeneration of the anterior horn cells of the peroneal nerves, *M. dystrophy.* A group of conditions also known as myopathies in which there is degeneration of groups of muscles without apparent nerve involvement.

Mutant. An individual possessing characteristics due to a genetic change.

Mutation. Genetic change, producing change in the individual of the species.

Myasthenia. Debility of the muscles.

Myasthenia gravis. A progressive loss of power in groups of muscle. Relieved by injections of prostigmine and surgical removal of the thymus gland.

Mycobacterium. A gram positive genus of bacteria. *M. leprae* causes leprosy and *M. tuberculosis*, tuberculosis.

Mycosis. Disease caused by fungus.

Mydriasis. Increase in the size of the pupil of the eye.

Mydriatics. Drugs which dilate the pupil of the eye, *e.g.* atropine, homatropine.

Myelin. Medullary sheath of a nerve.

Myelitis. Inflammation of the spinal cord.

Myelocyte. Bone marrow cell.

Myelogram. Radiograph of the spinal cord.

Myeloid. Of the marrow. *M. tissue.* Tissue giving rise to the cellular elements of the blood, *viz.* red cells, white cells and platelets.

Myeloma. Neoplasm of plasma cells.

Myelosclerosis. Replacement of bone marrow by fibrous tissue.

Myocardial. Pertaining to the muscle of the heart.

Myocarditis. Inflammation of the muscular tissue of the heart. Often follows acute rheumatism.

Myocardium. The heart muscle.

Myoglobin. A specialized haemoglobin found in muscle which has slightly different dissociation characteristics from that in the blood so that oxygen is transferred from the blood to the muscle.

Myoma. Any tumour composed of muscular tissue.

Myomectomy. Removal of a myoma: usually referring to a fibroid from the uterus.

Myope. A shortsighted person. *Myopic*, pertaining to shortsightedness.

Myopia. Shortsightedness: corrected by wearing a biconcave lens.

Myosarcoma. A malignant tumour of muscle.

Myosin. Protein found in muscle.

Myosis. Contraction of the pupil of the eye.

Myositis. Inflammation of a muscle. *M. ossificans.* May follow stretching of an injured muscle. Its fibres and haematoma are replaced by cancellous bone. The condition can be prevented by resting the injured muscle.

Myotics. Drugs which cause the pupil to contract. *e.g.* eserine. *Syn.* meiotics, miotics.

Myotomy. Cutting through a muscle.

Myringa. The tympanic membrane of the ear.

Myringitis. Inflammation of the tympanic membrane of the ear.

Myringotomy. Incision of the tympanic membrane of the ear, performed when the presence of the pus is suspected in the middle ear.

Myxoedima. Syndrome due to hypothyroidism and characterized by dry atrophic skin, swelling of the limbs and face and retardation both physical and mental. The metabolic rate is diminished and the patient dislikes the cold intensely.

Myxoma. Tumour of connective tissue containing mucoid material.

Naegele's obliquity. Tilting of the fetal head towards one or other shoulder as it enters the brim of the pelvis; by this attitude a slightly smaller transverse diameter of the head is presented to the brim.

Naevus. A birthmark due to a mass of dilated veins of arteries, usually very tiny ones.

Nail, Horny plate found at the tip of finger or toe.

Napkin rash. Inflammation of the 'napkin area' in a baby. Caused by alkalis, dampness, friction or infection. The nappies should not be washed in detergents as this is a frequent cause of the rash.

Narcissism. An abnormal love for oneself; named after Narcissus, who fell in love with the reflection of himself.

Narco-analysis. In psychotherapy, the patient is made to talk freely, bringing repressed matter to consciousness after having had an injection of a sedative drug.

Narcolepsy. A condition characterized by sudden attacks of sleep occurring repeatedly during the day.

Narcosis. A state of unconsciousness produced by the use of narcotics.

Narcotic. A drug which produces unconsciousness, *e.g.* paraldehyde, the barbiturates.

Nares. The nostrils.

Nasal. Relating to the nose.

Nasopharyngeal. Pertaining to the naso-pharynx.

Nasopharynx. The space between the posterior nares, the base of the skull, the soft palate, the upper end of the oesophagus, and the epiglottis.

Natural childbirth. A school of the opinion concerning childbirth which advocates the minimum of medical interference with the process of delivery.

Nausea. A feeling of sickness.

Navel. The umbilicus, the point of connection of the umbilical cord.

Navicular. The boat-shaped tarsal bone.

Nebula. A cloud or mist. Term applied to filmy corneal opacities.

Nebulae. Plural of nebula. Used to describe spray of very fine particles used, for example, to facilitate absorption of inhaled substances.

Neck. Narrow part near the end of an organ.

Necrobiosis. Death of tissue. *Red n.* A type of degeneration occuring in a fibroid of the uterus if pregancy takes place. After labour, the fibroid can recover its vitality.

Nematodes. Worms including round worms, threadworms and eelworms. Some of these are parasitic to man, *e.g.* hookworm.

Neoplasm. A tumour. An abnormal local multiplication of some type of cell. A neoplasm may be either *benign* if it shows no tendency to spread, or *malignant* if the growing cells infiltrate surrounding tissues and invade other parts of the body.

Nephrectomy. Removal of a kidney.

Nephritis. Inflammation of the kidney. The term nephritis is used to describe a large number of widely differing conditions affecting this organ.

Nephroblastoma. Wilms, tumour. A neoplasm of the kidney which occurs in children.

Nephrocalcinosis. A complication of hyperparathyroidism in which calcium becomes deposited in the renal tubes.

Nephrocapsulectomy. Operation to remove the kidney capsule.

Nephrography. X-ray examination of the kidney.

Nephrolithiasis. Stone in the kidney.

Nephrolithotom. Removal of a stone from the interior of the kidney.

Nephroma. Tumour of the kidney.

Nephron. A unit of the kidney. It consists of a glomerulus, with the secreting part of its tubule. One kidney has about a million nephrons.

Nephropexy. Stitching a movable kidney into a firm position.

Nephroptosis. Downward displacement of the kndney.

Nephrosis. Chronic progressive, degenerative disease of the renal tubes.

Nephrostomy, Surgical opening into the kidney to drain it.

Nephrotic syndrome. Degenerative disease of renal tubules characterized by heavy proteinuria, with reduction of plasma protein and oedema. Prognosis variable.

Nephrotomy. Cutting into the kidney.

Nephro-ureterectomy. Operation to remove both kidney and ureter.

Nerve. A bundle of fibres, conveying the impulses of movement and sensation to and from the organs.

Nerve root. Each spinal nerve arises from the spinal cord by two roots; the dorsal root carries the sensory fibres and the ventral root the motor fibres.

Nervous. Pertaining to the nerves. May also mean anxious and excited.

Neuralgia. Pain in the distribution of a nerve. *e.g. trigeminal n.* Severe pain in the distribution of the trigeminal nerve. Severe pain in the distribution of the trigeminal nerve. Sciatica is neuralgia of the sciatic nerve distribution. The cause may be irritation of the nerve by some bony structure or a tumour, but frequently the cause cannot be ascertained. For intractable pain interruption of the sensory fibres of the nerve is often helpful.

Neurofibromatosis. Von Reckling-hausen's disease. Generalized distribution within the body of neurofibromata.

Neuroglia. connective tissue cells of the central nervous system are collectively known as glia. Neuroglia are cells with long fibrous processes which are derived from embryonic nervous tissue and are closely related to schwann cells; their exact supportive function is not known. Microglia are similar to macrophages.

Neurosis. A disorder of mental function whereby patients ar abnormally emotionally vulnerable but retain external reality; cf. psychosis. Neuroses include behaviour disorders such as hysterical and obsessive compulsive reactions and disturbances of 'affect', as for example, in anxiety states.

Neurosurgery. Surgery of peripheral and central nervous system.

Neurosyphilis. Involvement of the central nervous system by syphilis.

Neutropaenia. Insufficiency of neutrophil polymorphonuclear leucocytes in the blood.

Neutrophil. Predilection for neutral dyes. *i.g.* not acidophil or basophil. Term used to describe the majority of polymorphonuclear leucocytes which do not demonstrate any characteristically staining granules in their cytoplasm, cf. basophil, eosinophil.

Nicotine, epoisoning. Result of over-indulgence in smoking due to an alkloid in tobacco leaves. Cardinal features are the paralysis of autonomic ganglia and constriction of coronary arteries.

Nicotinic acid, Pellagra-preventing factor of vitamin B complex.

Nictitation, Involuntary blinking of the eyelids.

Nidation Implantation.

Niemann-Pick's disease. A lipoid storage disease in which lecithin is deposited. An inherited defect of phospholipid metabolism which leads to widespread deposition of lecithin in the tissues. It is associated with mental retardation.

Nipple. Small eminence in the centre of each breast.

Nipple shields. Covering of glass or india-rubber put on the nipples to protect Them when they are sore.

Nissl's granules. Granular substances found in the cell body of a neuron.

Nobecutane. Resinous spray used to form a covering over wounds.

Nocturia. Passing urine at night. May be a symptom of cardiac failure.

Nocturnal. At night. *N. enuresis.* Bedwetting during sleep.

Nose. The organ of smell and used for warming, filtering and moistening the air breathed in.

Nosology. Science of the classification of diseases.

Nostalgia. Home sickness, or a yearning for the past.

Nostrils. The anterior apertures of the nose.

Notch. Indentation.

Notifiable. A term applied to certain cases of disease and other occurrences which must be made known to the District Medical Officer, *e.g.* smallpox, tuberculosis, typhoid fever, dysentery, food poisoning, acute poliomyelities, diphtheria, measles, whooping cough, etc.

Nucleus. *Pl. nuclei.* (1) Of cell, the spherical body containing the chromosomes. *See* CELL. (2) Of brain. demarcated mass of cell bodies. e.g. basal nuclei.

Nucleus pulposus. A pulpy mass in the centre of the intervertebral discs. May become prolapsed into the spinal canal causing pressure on the cord and spinal nerves.

Nullipara. A woman who has never had a child.

Nummulated, Resembling a coin; applied to a form of expectoration sometimes seen in pulmonary tuberculosis.

Nutation. Involuntary nodding of the head.

Nutrient. Nourishing. *N. foramen,* opening in a bone for the nourishing vessels.

Nutrition. Science of feeding.

Nyctalopia. A state of the eyes which causes vision to be worse at night than during the day.

Nyctophobia. Abnormal fear of darkness.

Nymphae. Labia minora.

Nymphomania. Excessive sexual desire in females.

Nystagmus. Involuntary oscillations of the eyeball; sometimes congenital; sometimes a symptom of brain disease, ocular affection, or lesion in the internal ear.

O Signs. Signs seen in a patient about which he may not complain.

Obsession. An idea of which the patient cannot rid himself. Minor obsessions are common in perfectly healthy people; but long- standing obsessions are especially frequent in the mentally ill.

Obsessive compulsive neurosis. Mental disorder in which the outstanding feature is a feeling of compulsion to act in a way which the patient realizes to be absurd.

Obstetric. Pertaining to the practice of midwifery.

Obstetrician. Doctor who practises obstetrics.

Occlusive theraphy. The patient is encouraged to use the lazy eye ball covering the good eye.

Occult blood. Not visible to naked eye. Term used to describe blood passed in faeces in such small amounts that no dark colour is present. This blood can only be demonstrated by the occult blood test.

Occupational therapist. One who practises occupational therapy.

Occupational therapy. Any occupation given to a patient to help in his recovery, both mentally and physically.

Ocular. Relating to the eye.

Oculist. An eye specialist.

Oedema. Abnormal amount of fluid in the tisues causing a puffy swelling. The fluid tends to collect in the dependent parts, e.g. oedema of the ankles.

Oesophageal. Pertaining to the oesophagus. *O. varices.* Varicose veins in the lower part of the oesophagus resulting from hypertension in the hepatic portal system which occurs in cirrrhosis of the liver.

Oesophagectomy. Resection of the oesophagus.

Oesophagitis. Inflammation of the oesophagus, especially *reflex o.*, due to hiatus hernia when stomach acid regurgitates into the lower part of the oesophagus causing damage and inflammation of the wall.

Oesophagoscope. An instrument for viewing the interior of the oesophagus.

Oesophagostomy. An artificial opening is made into the oesophagus.

Oesophagus. The canal which runs from the pharynx into the stomach.

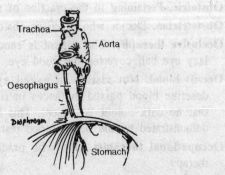

The oesophagus

Oestradiol. Hormone contained in Graafian follicles. Administered in oestrogen deficiency.

Oestrogen, or oestrogenic substance or hormone. Any substance, usually a steroid, capable of producing genital tract changes characteristic of the follicular phase of the menstrual cycle: an oestrogen is secreted by the ovaries. Oestrogens are also produced by the placenta during pregnancy and by the adrenal cortex. The female secondary sexual characteristics are under the influence of oestrogens.

Ointment. A soft application to promote healing, usually consisting of a base impregnated with some drug.

Olivary body. An oval mass of grey matter behind the anterior pyramid of the medulla oblongata.

Omentocele. hernial sac ocntaining omentum.

Omentopexy. Fixation of the omentum.

Omentum. A fold of the peritoneum. The *great o.* is suspended from the greater curvature of the stomach and hangs in front of the gut. The *lesser o.* passes from the lesser curvature of the stomach to the transverse fissure of the liver.

Oocyte. An ovum before it has left the Graafian follicle.

Oogenesis. The production of ova in the ovary.

Oophorectomy. Removal of an ovary.

Oophoritis. Inflammation of an ovary.

Oophoron. That portion of the ovary which produces the ova. Or the ovary itself.

Oophorosalpingectomy. Removal of the ovary and its associated Fallopian tube.

Opacity. Want of transparency, cloudiness.

Opaque, Not transparent.

Opening snap. Adventitious heart sound which often

precedes the mid-diastolic murmur of mitral stenosis.

Ophthalmia. Inflammation of the eye. The term is applied especially to severe inflammations of the conjunctiva. There is an acute infectious form which occurs in epidemics, especially in schools and military camps.

Ophthalmia neonatorum. Severe inflammation of the eyes in the newly born, due to gonorrhoeal or septic infection of the conjunctiva during he passage of the head through the vagina. When due to the gonococcus it responds to intensive treatment with penicillin, locally and by injection.

Ophthalmitis. Inflammation of the eye.

Ophthalmologist. A surgeon specializing in diseases of the eye.

Ophthalmology. The study of diseases of the eye.

Ophthalmoplegia. Paralysis of the muscles of the eye.

Ophthalmoscope. A small instrument, fitted with a lens, used to examine the interior of the eye.

Ophthalmotonometer. Instrument to measure the intra-ocular tension of the eye.

Optic. Relating to the sight. *O. atrophy*. Degeneration of the optic nerve.

Optic chiasma. The crossing of the fibres of the optic tract.

Optic disc. The point where the optic nerve enters the eye. This point is insensitive to light and is known as the blind spot.

Optician. Maker of optical instruments.

Optics. The dtudy of the properties of light.

Optimum. The best possible in the particular circumstances.

Optometry. Measurement of visual powers.

Oral. Pertaining to the mouth.

Orbicularis. A name given to a muscle which encircles an orifice. *e.g. O. oris*, around the mouth.

Orbit, The bony cavity in the skull which holds the eye.

Orchidectomy. Removal of one or both testicles. Castration.

Orchidopexy. the bringing down of an imperfectly descended testicle into the scrotum and fixing it there by sutures.

Orchiepididymitis. An inflamed epididymis and testicle.

Orchis. Testicle.

Orchitis. Inflammation of the testicles.

Organ. A part constructed to exercise a special function.

Orthopaedic. Surgery relating to the correction of deformities of the skeleton.

Orthopnoea. Breathlessness, the patient gaining relief only in an upright position.

Orthoptics. Term applied to correcting defective vision in a squint by exercise. etc.

Orthostatic. Pertaining to or caused by standing upright.

Osiander's sign. Sign appears during first three months of pregnancy when vaginal pulsation is felt.

Osler's nodes. Small tender inflamed areas in the skin particularly in the pulp of the fingers due to small emboli; occurs in bacterial endocarditis.

Osmotic fragility test. Method of determinining the fragility of red blood cells.

Osmotic pressure. Pressure required to prevent the passage of water by osmosis. The osmotic pressure depends on the number of solute molecules in solution.

Ossicle. A small bone. Name applied to the tiny bones of the middle ear.

Ossification. Hardening into bone.

Osteitis, Inflammation of bone. *O. fibrosa,* a disease of bone caused by an adenoma of the parathyroid glands. As the result of excessive secretion calcium is absorbed from the bones into the blood.

Osteoarthritis. Diesease due to excessive wear and tear on joint surfaces. Affecting chiefly weight-bearing joints, late in life, and resulting in pain, especially at night, deficient movement, and deformity.

Osteoarthropathy. Damage or disease affecting bones and joints.

Osteoarthrotomy. Excision of joint and neighbouring bone.

Osteoclasts. Multinucleated cells which break down the calcified bone matrix, Remodelling of bone by the combined activity of osteoclasts and osteoblasts occurs continuously during bone growth.

Osteopathy. A school of thought ascribing many diseases to structural derangement of skeletal parts and treating same by manipulation of joints. Term can also mean any bone disease.

Osteopetrosis. *See* MARBLE BONE DISEASE.

Osteophony. Conduction of sound by bone.

Osteophyte. A bony outgrowth or nodosity; occurs in osteoarthritis.

Otitis. Inflammation of the ear. *O. externa.* Inflammation of the skin of the external ear. *O. interna.* Inflammation of the inner ear affecting the organs of balance. *O. media.* Inflammation of the middle ear.

Otologist. Ear specialist.

Otology. Study of diseases of the ear.

Otophone. Eartrumpet.

Otorrhoea. A purulent discharge from the ear.

Ovarian cyst. Cyst of the ovary; may be developmental or associated with ovarian tumour.

Ovaries. Two small oval bodies situated on either side of the uterus; the female organs in which ova are formed. They are also endocrine glands.

Ovariectomy. Oophorectomy. Surgical removal of ovary.

Ovariotomy. The operation of cutting into an ovary.

Oviduct. The Fallopian tube between the ovary and the womb, conveying the ova.

Ovulation. The development and discharge of ova from the ovary.

Ovum. The egg cell produced in the female ovary.

Oxyhaemoglobin. Haemoglobin in which oxygen is in combination -as the in red cells of the blood.

Oxyntic. Term applied to cells secreting hydrochloric acid in the stomach.

Oxytocics. Drugs used to induce labour and to promote uterine contractions, *e.g.* pituitrin.

Oxytocin. The oxytocic hormone of the posterior lobe of the pituitary gland.

Oxyuriasis. Infection with oxyuris vermicularis.

Oxyuris vermicularis. Threadworm found in the rectum and large intestine, especially in children.

Ozaena. Form of atrophic rhinitis.

Ozone. O^3. An oxidizing agent sometimes used as a disinfectant.

Ozonic ether. A solution of hydrogen peroxide in ether.

Pacemaker. Initiator of heart impulse at sinuatrialnode. An electrical stimulator can be fitted surgically.

Pachymeningitis. Inflamation of the dura mater, with thickening of the membrane.

Pacini's corpuscles. Specialized sensory receptors which register pressure and to some extent vibration. They are situated in the deeper connective tissues of the skin and consist of nerve endings surrounded by concentric lamellae of fibrous tissue.

Pack. (1) Moistened material applied to a patient. (2) Thressing and/or instruments required for a sterile procedure, sterilised in a paper container.

Paediatrician. Specialist in diseases of children.

Paediatrics. The science or study of diseases of children.

Paget's disease. (1) Of bone, osteitis deformans, is a disorder of unknown cause which usually affects a number of bones to a greater or lesser extent. (2) Of nipple, Eczema of the nipple associated with underlying duct carcinoma of the breast.

Painter's colic. Lead poisoning.

Palate. The roof of the mouth.

Palatoplegia. Paralysis of soft palate.

Palliative. A medicine which relieves but does not cure.

Pallidectomy. Operation used in Parkinson's disease to decrease the activity of art of the lentiform nucleus in the base of the brain.

Pallidotomy. Operation performed to relieve tremor in Parkinson's disease. Fibres from the cerebral cortex are severed.

Palm. The hollow or flexor surface of the hand.

Palpation. Examination by the hand.

Palpitation. Rapid throbbing of the heart, producing conciousness of the heart's action.

Panarthritis. Generalized inflammation of joint structures.

Pancarditis. Generalized inflammation of the heart.

Pancreas. Sweetbread. A gland situated in the mesentery in

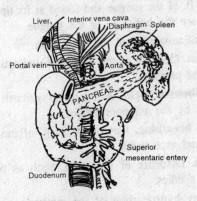

The pancreas

relation to the doudenum and crossing the mid-line of the body. It secretes an alkaline mixture of digestive enzymes through the pancretic duct into the doudenum when stimulated by the hormone *secretin*. It also contains groups of cells which secrete insulin into the blood.

Pandemic. A widely sperad epidemic.

Panhypopituitarism. Simmond's disease. Deficient secretion of all of the anterior pituitary hormones with additional secondary reduction in production of hormones by the thyroid and adrenal cortex.

Panophthalmia, panophthalmitis. Generalized inflammation of the eyeball.

Panotitis. Inflammation of the middle and internal ear.

Papanicolaou stain. Stain frequently employed for the examination of vaginal smears.

Papilla. Plu. papillae. (1) A small nipple-shaped eminence. (2) The optic disc. *Circumvallate papillae.* These are found at the root of the tongue. *Filiform papillae.* The common P. of the tongue and found at its tip. *Fungiform papillae* are the broad p. of the tongue.

Papillitis. Inflammation of the optic disc.

Papilloedema. Oedema of the optic disc indicative of raised intracranial pressure.

Para-aminobenzoic acid. A bacterial growth factor antagonized by the sulphanilamides.

Paradoxical breathing. Part of the lung inflates during expiration and vice versa.

Paraesthesia. Disorder of sensation, such as tingling and pins and needles.

Paraffin. Any hydrocarbon of the methane series. Liquid paraffin is refined petroleum. Soft paraffin is used as a lubricating jelly. Hard paraffin in paraffin wax. P. *gauze dressing.* Gauze impregnated with soft yellow paraffin jelly; used for burns and wounds.

Paraformaldehyde. Used to fumigate closed spaces, also

for sterilization of catheters and instruments when kept in an air- tight container filled with paraformaldehyde.

Paralysis. Loss of power of movement or of sensation. Usually due to a lession in the nervous system. *Spastic p.* is due to a lesion of upper motor neurones. *Flaccid p.* is the result of an injurty to lower motor neurones. *Infantile paralysis* is another name for poliomyelitis.

Paralytic ileus. Intestinal obstruction due to paralysis of the muscles of peristalsis, often caused by peritonitis.

Parasite. Any living thing which lives on or in another organism.

Parasympathetic system. Part of the autonomic nervous system acting in opposition to the sympathetic system. e.g. parasympathetic action causes constriction of the pupil, stimulation of the gut, etc.

Parathormone. The hormone of the parathyroid glands.

Parathyroid. Small endocrine glands which control calcium and phossphate metabolism. They are usually four in number and they are situated in the vicinity of the thyroid gland.

Paratyphoid. An infectious disease resembling typhoid fever and caused by an organism not identical with but closely allied to the bacillus of typhoid.

Parenteral treatment. Theraphy by drugs given by routes other than the alimentary tract.

Paresis. A partial paralysis.

Parietal. The two bones which from the crown and sides of the cranium.

Parity. The number of children a woman has borne.

Parkinson's disease. Also called paralysis agitans. A chronic disease of later life, showing tremors, rigidity of joints and muscles, a mask-like expression and walking with a tendency to fall forwards.

Paronychia. Whitlow; inflammation and abscess at the end of a finger near the nail.

Parotid. Near the ear; applied to a salivary gland under the ear.

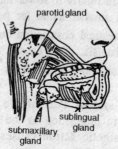

The parotid gland

Parotitis. Inflammation of the parotid gland. (1) Mumps. (2) Spread of infection from a septic mouth.

Paroxysm. A sudden temporary attack.

Paroxysmal nocturnal dyspnoea, Attacks of breathlessness occurring at night due to pulmonary oedema resulting from left ventricular failure.

Paroxysmal tachycardia. Is due to the regular and rapid discharge of impulses from ectopic focus in the atrial walls of the heart. The focus thus replaces the sinuatrial node as the cardiac pacemaker and drives the heart at a rate of about 180 beats per nimute. Attacks may last anything from a minute to several days.

Parturient. In the condition of giving or being just about to give birth to a child. The *parturient canal* is the passage traversed by the fetus during birth, from the brim of the pelvis to the vulva.

Parturition. The act of giving birth to a child.

Paschen bodies. Minute bodies containing the virus of smallpox.

Pasteurella. Group of bacilli causing bubonic and pneumonic plague. Carried by rats to man.

Pasteurization. Method of sterilization of fluids introduced by Pasteur which involves heating for 30 minutes at 70 °C.

Patellar bursae. The bursae around the patella. Inflammation of the prepatellar bursa used to be called housemaid's knee, as it occurs after much kneeling.

Patellectomy. Operation to excise the patella.

Patent. Open. P. *ductus arteriosus.* Failure of the ductus arteriosus to close at birth. P. *foramen ovale.* Failure of closure of the foramen ovale.

Pathogenesis. The origin and progress of disease.

Pathogenic. Capable of causing disease.

Pathological. Relating to pathology. Morbid, abnormal.

Pathology. The study of disease, particularly regarding the changes in the tissues resulting from disease.

Paul-Bunnell test. A serological test for glandular fever (infective mononucleosis).

Paul's tube. Glass drainage tube used to drain the bowel.

Pearson bed. Special bed for nursing fractures.

Peau d'orange. Orange-skin appearance of skin overlying carcinoma of the breast which is caused by obstruction to superficial lymphatics.

Petin. A polysacharide found in fruit.

Pectoral. Relating to the chest. P. *muscles* are on the anterior surface of chest.

Pectus. The thorax, chest.

Pedicle needle An instrument for passing a ligature round the pedicle of a tumour.

Pediculosis, Infestation with lice.

Pediculus. The louse, a parasite infesting the hair and skin. *P. capitis* infests the head; *P. corporis*, the body and clothing; *P. pubis*, the pubic hair. These three varieities are different in shape and size.

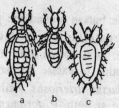

Pediculus (magnified): A = Capitis
B = Corporis C = Pubis

Pel-Ebstein's fever. A regularly remitting fever which sometimes occurs in Hodgkin's disease.

Pellagra. A nutritional disease especialy prevalent in southern Europe and in the southern United States of America. It is marked in the initial stages by recurring redness and exfoliation— resembling sunburn — of the hands and face. There may be glossitis, diarrhoea and peripheral neuritis, and mental changes. The anti-pellagra factor is vitamin B^6.

Pellet. A small pill, esp. those used as implants.

Pelvic exenteration. Operative removal of organ from pelvis.

Pelvimetry. Measurement of pelvic dimensions.

Pelvis. The bony cavity composed of the hips and the lower bones of the spine and holding the bowels, bladder and organs of generation.

Pemphigus. Disease characterized by the formation of large blisters on the skin and mucous membranes.

Penis. The male organ of coition containing the urethra.

Pentagastrin. A gastric acid stimulant used to test the secretion of the stomach.

Pepsin. An enzyme which breaks down proteins in acid solution to form peptides (*peptidase*). It is secreted in the stomach with hydrochloric acid.

Perception. An awareness. Receiving impressions through the senses.

Pericardial adhesions. Fibrosis of the pericardium which may follow pericarditis in which the two layers of the pericardium becomes stuck together.

Pericarditis. Inflammation of the pericardium; apt to follow on cases of acute rheumatism, typhoid, Bright's disease pneumonia or pyaemia.

Pericardium. The membranous sac which holds the heart. *Adherent* p. Rheumatic carditis is often followed by an adherent pericardium, especially after a pericarditis. This condition interferes with the free action of the heart.

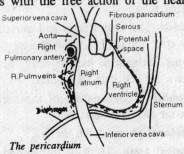

The pericardium

Perilymph. Clear fluid in the osseous labyrinth of the ear.

Perimetry. Measurement of visual field.

Perinatal mortality rate. The number of stillbirths and deaths in the first week of life of babies weighting more than 1,000g at birth per 1,000 births.

Perineorrhaphy. Operation for repairing a perineum ruptured during labour.

Perinephric. Round about the kidney. *P. abscess*, a collection of pus in the tissues round the kidney.

Perineum. The region of the pelvic floor, anterior to the anus.

Periodonatal membrane. Ligament attaching the tooth to the walls of its socket. *P. disease*. Annormalities of the supporting structures of the teeth.

Periosteotome. Knife used to incise the periosteum.

Periosteum. The membrane covering a bone.

Periostitis. Inflammation of the periosteum.

Peripheral. Relating to the circumference or outer surface. *P. neuritis.* Inflammation of the peripheral nerves.

Periproctitis. Inflammation of tissue around the rectum or anus.

Perisalpingitis. Inflammation of peritoneum covering the uterine tube.

Peristalsis. The contractions and movements of the alimentary tract forcing on the contents.

Peritomy. Incision of the conjuctiva near the margin of the cornea for the cure of pannus.

Perityphlitis. Inflammation of the peritoneum around the caecum and appendix.

Periurethral. Around the urethra.

Permanent teeth. Teeth of the second dentition.

Permanganate of potash. Antiseptic and disinfectant. Care should be imployed in its use, as it is poisonous in crystal state.

Pernicious. Tending to a fatal issue. *P. anaemia.* Anaemia resulting from cyanocobalamin (vitamin B^{12}) deficiency.

Perseveration. A recurring idea, feeling or way of action from which the patient finds it difficult to escape.

Personality. The make-up of a person with all his individual characteristic, both inherited and acquired.

Perspiration. Sweat, which is excreted through the pores of the skin.

Pertussis. Whooping cough; an infectious spasmodic cough, common in childhood. The cough ends with a whoop and sometimes causes an attack of vomiting. The disease runs its course in four to eight weeks' time. A serious disease in young children who may be vaccinated against it. Caused by haemophilus pertussis.

Pesticide. Term used to describe a substance that kills harmful or disease carrying insects or oragnisms.

Pestilence. Virulent infectious epidemic disease.

Petechiae, Small red spots on the skin formed by effusion of blood.

Peyer' patches. Small glands situated on the surface of the ileum and jejunum. Seat of ulceration in typhoid and paratyphoid fever.

pH. Scale of values denoting the hydrogen ion concentration of solutions and thus their alkalinity or acidity. Values below 7 are acid and those above 7 are alkaline.

Phaeochromocyte. One of two cell types present in the adrenal medulla and in the sympathetic ganglion.

Phaeochromocytoma. Tumour of phaeochromocytes usually arising in the adrenal medulla and producing hypertension, hyperglycaemia and irregularity of cardiac rhythm.

Phagocytes. The polymorphonuclear white cells of the blood, so called from their property of being able to ingest and destroy micro-organisms of disease which may be circulating in the blood or attacking the tissues.

Phagocytosis. The process of enveloping and absorbing a hostile germ by a phagocyte.

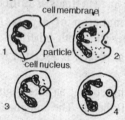

Phagocytosis

Phalanges. The small bones of the fingers and toes.

Pharmaceutical. Pertaining to drugs.

Pharmacology. A study of drug action.

Pharmacopoeia. An authorized handbook of drugs.

Pharmacy. (1) The science of preparing and mixing medicines or drugs (2) The place where drugs are prepared and distributed.

Pharyngeal. Pertaining to the pharynx. *P. pouch.* Diverticulum in the wall of the pharynx which may form between the two portions of the inferior constrictor muscle of the pharynx.

Pharynx. The musculo-membranous sac at the back of the mouth leading to the oesophagus and to the larynx.

Phenylalanine. Essential amino-acid.

Phenylketonuria. Genetically determined error of metabolism in which there is an inability of the liver to convert phenylalanine to tyrosine. Instead phenylalanine is broken down to phenylpyruvic acid which is excreted in the urine. There is associated mental deficiency.

Phelbitis. Inflammation of a vein, most commonly caused by the invasion of its coats by microorganisms. Associated with thrombosis, or coagulation of the blood in the vein.

Phelbolith. Calcified venous thrombus.

Phlebothrombosis. Thrombosis in veins, particularly the veins of the legs, due to prolonged haemostasis.

Phebotomus. Genus of small flies bringing disease such as kala-azar.

Phlebotomy. Bleeding a patient by opening a vein. venesection.

Phlegm. Sputum. Abnormal secretion of mucus from respiratory tract, the result of inflammation.

Phlegmasia. Inflammation. *P. alba dolens*, white leg; a form of phlebitis occurring sometimes after labour. The leg becomes swollen, white and tense, and is very painful.

Phlegmatic. Sluggish, dull.

Phlyctenule. Red pimples met with on surface of eye.

Phobia. Abnormal fear, *e.g.* cancerophobia, claustrophobia.

Phonation. The utterance of vocal sounds.

Phonocardiograph. Instrument recording heart sounds.

Phosphatase. Enzyme concerned in phosphate metabolism.

Phosphaturia. Excess of phosphates in the urine.

Phospholipid, Lipids containing phosphates, *e.g.* lecithin. They are particularly concerned in living systems with forming membranes.

Phosphonecrosis. Necrosis of the jaw, caused by inhaling phosphorus; occurs in certain trades, such as matchmaking, but is rare.

Phosphours. Poisonous non-metallic element the salts of which are used as 'nerve tonics'.

Photalgia. Pain caused by exposure to light.

Photobiology. The study of the effect of light on animal life.

Photophobia. Abnormal intolerance of light, a symptom of inflammation of the eyes.

Photosensitization. Tendency of tissues to react abnormally to light usually as the result of the presence in the tissues of certain chemicals which magnify the damaging effect of the incident radiation.

Phrenic. (1) Relating to the diaphragm. (2) Relating to the mind.

Phrynoderma. Follicular keratosis as occurs, for example, in vitamin. A deficiency.

Phthirus pubis. The pubic louse.

Phthisis, Consumption; tubercular disese of the lungs.

Physic. (1) The art of medicine. (2) Any medicinal preparation.

Physician. Qualified medical practitioner.

Physiological saline. A 0.9 per cent solution of sodium chloride in water. Formerly known as normal saline.

Physiology. The study of processes occurring in living systems.

Physiotherapy. Therapy by physical means, *i.e.* heat, light, electricity. massage, and exercise.

Physique. The from and constitution of the body.

Pia mater. The fine membrane surrounding the brain and spinal cord. The inner layer of meninges.

Pica, Morbid appetite. Craving for unnatural articles of food.

Pick's desease. (1) Disorder affecting serous membranes resulting in effusions in the peritoneum, pericardium and pleura. The cause is unknow. (2) Presenile dementia due to cerebral atrophy.

Pigment. An organic colouring matter. Abnormal pigmentation of the skin occurs in certain diseases, *e.g.* Addison's disease.

Piles, Enlarged veins about the anus; haemorrhoids.

Pilonidal, Containing hair as in some cysts. *P. sinuse.* Sinus containing hairs which may form in anal cleft and become infected, resulting in an abscess.

Pilosis. Abnormal growth of hair.

Pilula. A pill; abbreviation, *pil.*

Pineal body. The so-called 'third eye'. Develops from outgrowths of the forebrain, part of which forms an eye-like structure in the lamprey. In man it is a gland-like structure whose function is not determined.

Pink disease. Infantile acrodynia. A form of polyneuritis with particular involvement of the autonomic nervous system thought to be due to sencitivity to mercury from calomel containing teething powder.

Pinna. The outspread part of the ear.

Pituitary gland. Endocrine gland in the base of the skull; there are two lobes separated by a cleft. The *anterior lobe* secretes thyrotropic hormone, corticotrophic hormone (ACTH), gonadotrophic hormones (FSS,LH) growth hormone (GH) and prolactin. The posterior lobe secretes antidiuretic hormone and oxytocin.

Pityriasis rose. Skin disease characterized by scaly, erythematous macular eruption. Thought to be caused by a virus related to the measles virus.

Placebo. Medicine given to please the patient, but which in generally inactive.

Placenta. The after-birth; circular fleshlike substance through which the mother's blood nourishes the fetus; it is expelled from the womb after the birth of the child.

Placenta praevia. The placenta attached partially or totally to the lower uterine segment.

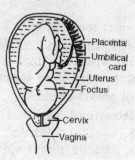

The placenta

Plague. An acute epidemic infectious disease cause by pasteurella pestis derive from infected rats and transmitted to man by fleas.

Plasma. The liquid in which the corpuscles of the blood are suspended.

Plasmodium malariae. Organism causing quartan malaria.

Plaster. Adhesive tape used for keeping dressings in position or for applying extension to a limb.

Plaster of Paris. Used for preparing bandages, in making splints to immobilize part of the body.

Plastic surgery. Restoration of tissue to its normal shape and appearance by operative means.

Platelets. Blood cells concerned with the clotting of blood. Normally number 200,000-500,000 per mm^3.

Pleocytosis. Increase of lymphocytes in cerebrospinal fluid.

Pleomorphism. Occurring in more than one form as with a crystal.

Plethora. Unhealthy repletion. An excess of blood.

Pleura. A thin membrane which covers each lung and lines the inner surface of the thoracic cavity.

Pleurisy. Inflammation of the pleura. There are three kinds; dry, with effusion, and empyema or purulent pleurisy.

Plezus, A network of vessels or nerves.

Plumbism. Lead poisoning.

Plummer-Vinson syndrome, Dysphagia occurring in patients with severe nutritional iron-deficiency anaemia.

Pneumococcus. A bacterium which causes pneumonia.

Pnemoconiosis. Fibrosis of the lungens caused by working in an atmosphere full of powdered grit and stone.

Pneumomycosis. Fungus disease of the lungs.

Pneumonectomy. Surgical removal of a lung.

Pneumonia, An infective disease charcterized by inflammation of the lungs. Double pneumonia, both lungs are diseased. *Hypostatic P.* is caused by lack of movement in a debilitated patient. May occure after operation or in the aged. *Lobar P.*, affecting one or more lobes of the lung.

Pneamonites. Inflammation of the lung.

Podalic version. A turning round of the fetus in utero, so the the breech presents in delivery.

Poikilocytosis. Variation in the form of the red blood cells.

Poison. A substance deleterious to the body if absorbed in toxic concentrations. The term is usually reseved for substances which are toxic in low concentrations, *e.g.* cyanide.

Poliomyelitis. Acute virus infection causing degeneration of the anterior horn cells of the spinal cord and conequent paralysis of the appropriate muscles.

Politzer's bag. An india-rubber bag with long tube and nozzle. Used for inflating the middle ear through the nose and Eustachian tube.

Polyarthritis. Inflammation of many joints.

Polya's operation. Operation for duodenal ulcer in which the stump of the stomach is anastomosed to the side of the jejenum.

Polycythaemia. (1) *Primary Polycythaemia.* Excessive production of erythropoietic cells. (2) *Secondary polycythaemia.* Increase in the number of red blood cells in the blood due to stimulation of the bone marrow, *e.g.* by anoxia at high altitudes or due to respiratory disease.

Polydactyly. The presence of supernumerary fingers or toes.

Polydipsia. Abnormal thirst.

Potymyositis. Weakness and wasting of muscles due to inflammation of unknown etiology.

Polyneuritis. Multiple neuritis.

Polyopia. Seeing multiple images of the same object.

Polyosteotic fibrous dysplasia, Albright's syndrome. A congenital disorder characterized by widespread osteitis fibiosa, segmental hyperpigmentation of the skin and, in girls, precocious sexual development.

Polyus. A small simple tumor occurring in the ear, nose, uterus or rectum.

Polyuria. Excessive flow of urine.

Pompholyx. A dermatitis with vesicles. A vesicular eruption occurring on the palms and soles. Probably a form of eczema.

Pons Varolii. That portion of the base of the brain which connects together the medulla oblongata, cerebrum and cerebellum. *See* BRAIN.

Pontine. Pertaining to the pons.

Popliteal. Pertaining to the popliteal space the area behind the knee.

Pore. A minute passage in the skin for perspiration; an opening between the molecules of a body.

Porphyria. Rare metabaolic disturbance which may cause mental damage in young children. There are convulsions, delirium, polyneuritis, etc.

Portal hypertension. Hypertension in the hepatic portal system usually resulting from cirrhosis of the liver.

Portal vein. The vein which conveys to the liver the blood circulating through the gastro-intestinal system and spleen.

Positive pressure ventilation. Air is pushed into the lungs either by manual method such as the Holger Nielson or by a mechanical devce.

Posset. In infant feeding, regurgitation of a feed.

Postclimacteric. After the menopause.

Postencephalitis. Condition which may remain after encephalitis.

Posterior chamber of eye. Small space lying behind iris and the lens and containing aqueous humor.

Posthumous. After death; a posthumous child is one born after the father's death.

Postmature. Infant born after the expected date of delivery.

Post Mortem. The opening and examining of a dead body.

Post-natal. Following birth.

Post-partum. After labour. *Post-partum hemorrhage* is excessive vaginal bleeding occurring either immediately after the birth of the baby or within a few days (secondary).

Pott's disease. Tuberculous disease of the spine, usually in children.

Pott's fracture. Fracture of the ankle with or without displacement of the joint mortice. Treatment dependent on the degree of injury.

Poultice. Soft and moist applications generally containing heat had applied to relieve pain, *e.g.* kaolin. Starch ponltices may be used in certain skin conditions.

Poupart's ligament. The ligament of the groin, stretching between the anterior superior spine of the ilium and the os pubis.

Precipate labour. Labour which is concluded in a time very much shorter than the average.

Precipitins. Protective substances in the blood which kill bacteria by 'precipitating' their protein content.

Precordium. The area of the chest over the heart.

Predigestion. Food is partially digested artificially before it is eaten as with a junket when rennet has curdled the milk.

Prefrontal. Lying in the anterior part of frontal lobe of the brain. *P. Leucotomy.*

Pregnancy. The state of being with child. Usual period 280 days.

Premature labour. Labour resulting in birth of premature baby, i.e. one weighing 2,500g or less.

Premedication. Drug given as a narcotic before a general anaesthetic.

Premenstrual. Before menstruation. *P. tension syndrome.* Syndrome consisting of tension, aniety, aches, depression and often accident-proness which occurs one a few days before menstrual period in some women. It is thought to be hormonal in origin.

Premolar. The two bicuspid teeth in each jaw which lie between the canine and the molars.

Premonitory. Giving warning beforehand.

Prenatal. Prior to birth, during the period of pregnancy.

Preparalytic. State before paralysis has occurred.

Prepuce. Loose skin covering the glans penis: foreskin.

Presbyopia. Long-sightedness due to inability of make lens of the eye convex by contraction of the ciliary muscles, *i.e.* failure of adaptation of the lens.

Prescription. A formula written by the physician to the dispenser. Consists of the heading, usually the symbol R meaning 'take', the names and quantities of the ingredients, the directions to the dispenser, the directions to the patient, the date and the signature.

Presentation. The part of the fetus which first engages or tends to engage in the pelvis is said to present, and the description of this part is the presentation.

Pressor. Substance causing blood pressure to rise.

Presystole. Period in the cardiac cycle before systole.

Priapism. Persistent erection of the penis.

Prickle cells. Epidermal cells furnished with radiating prosesses which connect with similar cells. P. Layer, the lowest stratum of the epidermis.

Prickly heat, Miliaria papillosa.

Primary focus. First site of infection in tuberculosis. Healing usually takes plase uneventfully.

Primary lesion. Original lesion from which others may arise.

Primary sore. Intitial site of infection in syphiles.

Primigravida. A woman pregnant for the first time.

Primipara. A woman who has borne one child.

Proctalgia. Pain about the rectum.

Proctectomy. Excision of rectum.

Proctitis. Inflammation of the rectum.

Proctocele. Prolapsed rectum.

Proctoclysis. Introduction into the rectum of fluid for absorption

Proctorrhaphy. Suturing of the rectum.

Proctoscope. An instrument for viewing the interior of the rectum.

Prodromal period, The period that elapses in an infectious disease between the appearance of the first symptoms and the development of the rash, *e.g.* in smallpox, 3 days.

Progeria. A condition in which premature senility is combined with infantilism.

Progesterone. The hormone of the corpus luteum which cause secretory changes in the uterine mucous membrane in pregnancy and during the menstrual cycle.

Progestogen. Substance having similar action to progesterone.

Proglottis. Segment of tapeworm.

Prognosis. The considered opinion as to the course of a disease.

Progressive muscular atrophy. Loss of power and wasting of muscles. Degenerative changes are found in the motor cells of the brain and anterior horns of the spinal cord.

Prolactin. Milk producing hormone of the anterior lobe of the pituitary.

Prolan. The original name given to the secretion of the

anterior lobe of the pituitary gland. *Prolan A* stimulates the Graafian follicle to ripen, and the production of oestrin. This is now called the follicle stimulating hormone or FSH. *Prolan B* stimulates the formation of the corpus luteum and the secretion of progesterone. This in now called luteinizing hormone or LH.

Prolapsed intervertebral disc. Slipped disc due to Prolapse of the central part of the cartilaginous intervertebral disc. *See* NUCLEUS PULPOSUS.

Proliferation, Reproduction. Cellgenesis.

Proprietary drug. A remedy with a registered trade name.

Proprioceptor, Sensory end organ which detects changes in position, *e.g.* of muscles or joints or fluid in the balancing apparatus of the inner ear.

Proptosis oculi. Protrusion of eyeballs.

Prostate. A gland associated with the male reproductive system. Its size and secretion are under the influence of androgens. Its function is not clear but it appears to supply supportive substances to the spermatozoa in the seminal vesicle.

Prostatectomy. Operation of removing the prostate gland. The operation may be suprapubic may be suprapubic when the bladder is first incised, or retropubic.

Prostatitis. Inflammation of the prostate gland.

Prosthesis. The replacement of an absent limb or organ by an artificial apparatus.

Protein. Very complex organic compound made up of a large number of amino-acids which are synthesized by living systems. There are 20 different amino-acids commonly found in proteins and these are arranged in different sequences which give the specific characteristics to the proteins.

Proteinuria. Protein in the urine.

Prothrombin. The substance which when activated by thrombokinase in the presence of calcium ions becomes thrombin.

Protoplasm. The living jelly-like substance which forms the main part of a cell. It is made up chiefly of water, proteins, and inorganic salts.

Proud flesh. Excessive granulation tissue in a wound.

Prurigo. A skin disease marked by irritating papules.

Pseudocyesis. Changes mimicking pregnancy but without a fetus.

Pseudohermaphrodite. The external sex organs are of different sexual type to the sex glands.

Pseudoplegia. Hysterical paralysis.

Pseudopodium. Temporary protrusion of cell serving as method of locomotion and phagocytosis.

Psittacosis. A virus disease found in parrots and other birds which is communicable to man. It manifests itself as an atypical pneumonia, which may be successfully treated with antibiotics.

Psoas. A large muscle attached above to the lumbar vertebrae and below to the femur. It flexes the femur on the trunk. *P. abscess.*

Psoriasis. Genetically determined abnormality of keratinization producing skin lesions consisting of raised, red scaly areas.

Psychiatrist. A doctor who specializes in psychiatry.

Psychiatry. The study and treatment of mental disorders.

Psycho-analysis. A method of treatment, based upon the theories of Freud, tracing nervous conditions to their antecedent causes,

Psychodynamics. Science of mental processes.

Psychologist. One who studies psychology but is not a doctor of medicine.

Psychology. The study of the mind.

Psychoneurosis. A functional mental disease.

Psychopath. A mentally deranged person.

Psychopathology. Study of the mechanism of mental disorders.

Psychosis. A severe mental disorder.

Psychosomatic, Relating to mind and body.

Psychotherapeutics, psychotherapy. Treatment of the mind. A term which includes any treatment for functional nervous disorders, *e.g.* by hypnotism, suggestion, psychoanalysis, etc.

Psychotic. Relating to a psychosis.

Pterygium. Mucous membrane growing on the conjunctiva and tending to grow on to the cornea.

Ptomaine. Posionous amines form bacterial decomposition of animal or vegetable matter.

Ptyalin. An enzyme which is present in saliva. It has the power of digesting starch. Now called salivary amylase.

Ptyalism. Excessive flow on saliva.

Puberty. The point in development when the reproductive organs become active.

Pubes. The two pubic bones. Also applied to the area above the bones.

Pudenda. The external genital organs.

Pudendal block. Method of anaesthesia in second stage of labour by injecting pudendal nerves transvaginally.

Puerperal fever. A continued fever following labour, and due to infection.

Puerperal insanity. Mental disorder following childbirth. A rare occurrence.

Puerperium. The period after a confinement until the uterus in involuted.

Pulmonary. Relating to the lungs. *P. stenosis.* Narrowing of the pulmonary valve of the heart. *P. valve.* The valve at the exit of the right ventricle into the pulmonary artery.

Pulsation. Bearing of the heart or of the blood in the arteries.

Pulse. Can be felt where an artery crosses a bone. It is usually taken at the wrist with three fingers on the radial artery. The pulse in health beats about 120 to the minute in infants; 80 in children: 60 to 70 in adults.

Pulsus alternans. The pulse is alternately strong and weak though regular in time.

Pupa. Second stage of insect development following the larval stage.

Pupil. the orifice in the centre of the iris.

Pupillary. Pertaining to the pupil.

Purgative. A medicine for causing evacuation of the bowels.

Purine diet, low. Prescribed for gout.

Purkinje cells. Nerve cells found in the cortex of the cerebellum.

Purpura. Red or purple spots or patches due to haemorrhages into the skin.

Pus. Matter. Consists of dead leucocytes, dead bacteria, cell debris and tissue fluid.

Pastule. A pinple containing pus.

Putrefaction. The rotting away of animal matter. Decomposition advanced to an offensive stage.

Pyaemia. The circulation of septic emboli in the blood stream causing multiple abscesses.

Pyarthrosis. Suppuration in a joint.

Pyelitis, Inflammation of the pelvis of the kidney. The organism is usually the *E. coli.* Now thought that it always includes renal substance and therefore is pyelonephritis.

Pyelography, The method to demonstrate kindneys, ureters and bladder, following intravenous injection of contrast medium opaque to x-rays. *retrograde. p.* The method to demonstrate kidneys and ureters following introduction of ureteric catheter into which contrast medium is injected.

Pyelodithotomy. Operation to remove a stone from the renal pelvis.

Pyelonephritis. Inflammation of the kidney and its pelvis.

Pylorectomy. Removal of the pyloric end of the stomach.

Pyloric stenosis. Narrowing of the pylorus. A condition found in infants, more commonly male than female.

Pyloroplasty. Operation for widening the contracted pylorus.

Pylorus. Region of the junction between the stomach and the duodenum.

Pyocolpos. Pus retained in the vagina.

Pyoderma. Any septic skin lesion.

Pyogenic. Producing, forming pus.

Pyometra. Pus retained in the uterus.

Pyonephrosis. Pus in the kidney.

Pyopericardium, Pus in the pericardium.

Pyopneumothorax, Pus and air in the pleural cavity.

Pyorrhoea. A flow of pus. Generally used as meaning the same as *pyorrhoea alveolaris,* a condition in which pus oozes out from the gums around the roots of the teeth. This is also known as Rigg's disease.

Pyosalpinx, Abscess in a Fallopian tube.

Pyrexia, Fever. Elevation of the body temperature. *Intermittent p.*, temperature high at night, below normal in the morning. *Remittent p.*, temperature high at night, down in morning, but never remaining normal. *Continuous p.*, with a variation of less than one degree Celsius.

Pyridoxin. Vitamin B^6 or adermin.

Pyrosis. A burning pain in the stomach with eructation; heart-burn.

Pyuria. Pus in the urine.

'Q' fever. Also known as Queensland fever. An acute disease resembling pneumonia and caused by Rickettsia burneti.

Quack. One who pretends to knowledge or skill which he does not possess.

Quadriplegia. Paralysis of both legs and arms.

Quadruple vaccine. Vaccine immunizing against tetanus, diphtheria, whooping cough and poliomyelitis.

Quarantine. A period of separation of infected persons or contacts from others, necessary to prevent the spread of disease.

Quartan. Refers to an intermittent fever rising and falling in period of 72 hours.

Quaternary ammonium compounds. Bactericides such as cetrimide, benzalkonium and domiphen.

Queckenstedt's test. To elicit the presence of spinal block, *e.g.* tumour. A lumbar puncture is performed. If the manometer shows no increase of intraspinal pressure when the jugular veins are pressed there is spinal block.

Quickening. Refers to the first perception of movement of the fetus in the womb, usually felt by the mother at the end of the fourth month.

Quinsy. A peritonsillar abscess, situated immediately outside the capsule of the tonsil.

Quintan. Remittent fever, which recurs every fifth day.

Quoddian. Recurring daily. Intermittent malarial fever.

Rabies. A specific infective disease: affects dogs chiefly, but may be transferred to human beings. *See* HYDROPHOBIA.

Rachitic. Due to rickets. A rachitic flat pelvis is a deformity of the pelvis due to rickets during childhood.

Radiation sickness. Diarrhoea and vomiting resulting from radiation.

Radioctive isotopes. Varieties of chemical elements which exhibit radioactivity.

Radiographer. Person trained to take x-rays.

Radiography. Science of examination by means of x-rays.

Radiologist. A doctor who has made a special study of radiology.

Radiology. The study of diagnosis by means of radiography.

Radiosensitive. Term applied to a structure, especially a tumour, responsive to radiotherapy.

Radiotherapy. The treatment of disease by radium, x-rays or other radioactive substances.

Radium. A disintegration product of uranium. It belongs to the group of radioactive elements; when isolated it is a white metal, but for medical purposes it is used as a compound, *i.e.* radium bromide for the production of radon, and radium sulphate for use in needles, plaques, etc, Radium disintegrates slowly, reaching half-strength in 1,690 years. Radium is a valuable thrapeutic agent, and is used chiefly to destroy malignant growths.

Radium rays. The rays emitted by radium are of three types, *i.e* alaha beta, and gamma rays.

Radius. The outer bone of the forearm, from the elbow to the wrist.

Radon. Radioactive gas derived from radium. *R seeds.* Sealed containers of radon.

Ramus. A branch; thus *ramus abdominalis*, branch from lumbar artery to abdominal walls. The term is also applied to branches of nerves.

Raphe. Fibrous junction between muscles.

Rapport. A good relatonship between two people.

Rash. Skin eruption.

Raspatory. A blunt instrument for dissecting tissues.

Rat-bite fever. Disease which occurs in China and japan. It is conveyed by the bite of an infected rat. The organism is known as the spirillum minus.

Raucous. Hoarse.

Ray fungus. The organism which causes actinomycosis.

Raynaud's diseases. Recurring vascular spasm of the extremities. The fingers become cold and white Occasionally dry gangrene occurs.

Recalcitrant. Resistant, esp. of a disease to its treatment.

Recall. Brining back a memory.

Receptacuium chyli. The lower expanded portion of the thoracic duct.

Receptor, Sensory nerve ending.

Recessive, (1) Tending to disappear. (2) An inhierited characteristic which does not appear in the next generation if the dominant gene is present.

Recipient. The person receiving blood by a transfusion.

Recrudescence,. Return of symptoms.

Rectocele. Prolapse of posterior vaginal wall. Strictly the term applies to any herniation of the rectum.

Rectopexy. Surgical procedure to fix a prolapsed rectum.

Rectum. The lower part of the large intestine from the colon to the anal canal. *See* BOWEL.

Red blood cell, These are the blood cells which contain haemoglobin (*erythrocytes*). There are about 5,000,000 in each mm^3 of blood and they carry nearly all the oxygen required by the body cells. Red blood cells are formed in the bone marrow, normally at a rate of about one million a second, and are notable for the absence of a nucleus in the mature state. They do not divide and have a lifetime of about 120 days when they arc destroyed in the spleen.

Red lotion. Astringant, contains sulphate of zinc.

Reduction. Replacing to a normal position, *e.g.* After fracture, dislocation or hernia.

Referred pain. Pain felt at a point quite different from the position of the affected part.

Reflex. Simplest form of nervous behaviour whereby a stimulus produces an almost instantaneous response due to an inborn nerve pathway, the *reflex arc*.

Regeneration. Renewal of damaged tissue such as regenerating nerve fibres.

Regurgitation. Flowing back. A backward flow of blood through defective values. Also used when fluid taken by the mouth regurgitates through the nose. This occurs with paralysis of the pharynx or soft palate, and may be one of the complications of diohtheria.

Reiter protein complement fixation test. One of the three ecreening tests for syphilis. The other two tests are the WR and the kahn test.

Reiter's syndrome. Urethritis combined with arthritis and conjunctivitis.

Relapse. A return of disease after convalescence has once begun.

Relapsing fever. Famine fever. A tropical disease caused by spirochaetes of the genus Borrelia.

Relaxant. Applied to drug used to relax muscle tone.

Relaixn. Ovarian secretion ehich softens the cervix and ligaments at child birth.

Renal. relating to the kidney. *R. calculus.* Stone in the kidney. *R threshold see* THRESHOLD.

Renin. Enzyme produced by the kidneys which may cause hypertension when there is a poor blood supply to the kidneys.

Rennin. A milk curdling enzyme present in the gastric juice.

Resectoscope. Instrument to view and remove pieces of tissue in transurethral prostatectomy.

Reserpine. An alkaloid from rauwolfia. The drug is a sedative which lowers blood pressure and slows the heart.

Respiration. Breathing. Rate should be in infants 50 to the minute in children 36, in adults 16. *Inverted r.* The pause is after inspiration instead of after expiration; noticed in babies with broncho-pneumonia.

Respirator. (1) Appliance worn over the mouth and nose to prevent the inhalation of poisonous gas. (2) Apparatus used to assist the muscles of respiration when paralysed, *e.g.* in poliomyelitis. There is a variety of types of these respirators.

Retching. Ineffectual efforts to vomit.

Retention. A holding back. Inability to void urine.

Reticulocyte. Immatureerythrocyte found in blood regeneration.

Reticulocytosis. Excessive reticulocytes found in the blood stream.

Reticulo-endothelial system. Special endothelial cells which are phagocytic and are found in spleen, lymph glands, liver and bone marrow. These cells aid in the destruction of red cells and form bilirubin from haemoglobin.

Reticuloses. A group of neoplastic disorders affecting the reticuloendothelial tissue and causing lymph node and splenic enlargement, *e.g.* Hodgkin's disease, lymphosarcoma.

Retina, The delicate inner coat of the eye between choroid and vitreous humour which is sensitive to light. It is the termination of the opticnerve upon which objects are focussed. *See* EYE.

Retractor. Instrument used to with draw structures obscuring the flied of operation.

Retrolental fibroplasia. The posterior part of the capsule of the lens of the eye becomes fibrosed and blindness may result. Found in premature babies who have been given too much oxygen.

Retroperitoneal. Behind the posterior layer of the peritoneum.

Retropharyngeal. Behind the pharynx. *R. Abscess,* a collection of pus behind the wall of the pharynx and anterior to the cervical vertebrae. An acute abscess may develop from inflammation of two glands near mid-line, a chronic one from cervical caries.

Reverdin's needle. A long handle with a curved needle at right angles. Used for deep work in pelvis. Needle is inserted beneath tissue required to be tied, threaded, then withdrawn, leaving ligature *in situ*. It can thus be tied.

Rhagades. A crack or fissure of skin causing pain; a term especially used of radiating scars at angle of mouth due to congenital syphilis.

Rheumatic. Pertaining to rheumatism. *R. fever.* Acute rheumatic fever is a disorder affecting connective tissue, particularly that of the heart and the joints. The cause is considered to be an allergic reaction to toxins from haemolytic streptococcus (Lancefield group A). *R. heart disease.* Chronic rheumatic heart disease is the result of severe damage and deformation of the heart due to rheumatic fever.

Rheumatism. General term covering diverse condition which have in common rather ill-defined pains of the muscles and joints.

Rheumatoid arthritis. A subacute or chronic form of arthritis. Gross changes occur in the joints leading to deformity and ankylosis.

Rheumatologist. One who studies rheumatic disease.

Rhinitis. Inflammation of the nose.

Rhinorrhoea. Discharge from the nose.

Rhinoscope. Nasal speculum.

Rhizodontropy. Dental term for crowning the root of a tooth.

Rhizotomy. Division of spinal nerve roots.

Rhodopsin. Visual purple contained in the retina.

Rhonchus. A rattling bronchial sound heard on auscultation.

Riboflavin. Part of vitamin B complex.

Ribonuclease. Enzyme which degrades RNA.

Ribonucleic acid. Chemical substance in animal cells. It is concerned in synthesis of protein.

Ribs. Long lateral bones enclosing the chest. The upper seven ribs on each side join the sternum by separate cartilages, and are called true ribs, the lower five ribs being termed false ribs. Of the latter, the upper three pairs are attached to the sternum by a common cartilage on each side; while the lower two ribs on each side are not attached to the sternum at all and are therefore called floating ribs.

Rice-water stools. Stools of cholera which look like water in which rice has been boiled.

Richter's hernia. Herniam which involves only a portion of the lumen of the intestine.

Rickets. Disease of childhood due to a diet lacking in vitamin D and lack of fresh air and sunshine. The child is fat but flabby, irritable; delay in walking and teething profuse sweats head large, anterior fontanelle open at 2 years, bossing of frontal bones pigeon breast beading of ribs, enlargement of epiphyses, deformities of long bones enlarged abdomen tendency to bronchitis and gastroenteritis.

Rickettsia. Microorganisms responsible for typhus and similar infections.

Rigor. Sudden feeling of cold accompanied by shivering which raises the body temperature above normal. Due to disorder of thermoregulatory center of the brain caused by toxins etc.

Rigor mortis. The stiffening of the body after death.

Ringer's solution. Physiological saline which includes, in addition to sodium, potassium, calcium, magnesium and some other ions normally present in extracellular fluid.

Ringworm. Also called tinea, fungus infection or dermatophytosis. Infection of the skin, hair or nails by various kinds of fungi. Some forms of ringworm as *microsporon audouini* only affect man; tinea verrucosum affects cattle but may be passed on to man affecting the scalp. *Microsporon felinum* affects dogs and cats and man secondarily. In body ringworm, *tinea circinata* there are spreading rings with blistery or scaling edges; in *tinea pedis* or athlete's foot, the skin between and behind the toes is specialy affected; onchomycosis is ringworm of the nails usually caused by trychophyton rubrum. Ringworm of the scalp may be caused by *microsporon audouini* or infection from cattle, dogs or cats. There are circular patches of dull colour. The hairs in the infected areas break off just above the scalp. Diagnosis is made with Wood's light and also microscope. Modern treatment is a course of griseofuivin by mouth for at least six weeks.

Rinne's test. A vibrating tuning-fork is placed on the mastoid process until no longer heard, then quickly put in front of the meatus; normally the vibration is still heard. The test is negative when obstruction exists in the external or middle ear.

Ripple mattress. Apparatus designed to reduce the incidence of pressure sore by rhythmically shifting weight of the patient from one area to the other by means of pumping air into linear compartments causing the mattress to 'ripple'.

Risus sardonicus. A convulsive grin, symptomatic of tetanus. **RNA.** *See* RIBONUCLEIC ACID.

Rodent ulcer. Basal cell carcinoma of skin.

Rods. Retinal organs giving night vision.

Romberg's sign. Inability to stand erect when the eyes are closed and the feet placed together; seen in tab's dorsalis.

Rotators. Muscles which cause circular movement.

Roughage. Cellulose part of food which gives bulk and aids peristalsis.

Round ligaments. Two thin cords passing from the uterus through the broad ligaments, and terminating in the canals of Nuck in the inguinal regions. When these are shortened for retroverted uterus, this is called Mackendrodt's operation.

Rovsing's sign. In appendicitis, pressure in the left iliac fossa will cause pain in the right iliac fossa.

Rubella. Also called German measles. A mild infectious disease caused by virus. Incuvation period 14-20 days infectiveity less than measles. There may be slight catarrh and fever and swelling of suboccipital glands. The rash begins on the face and spreads to the body and fades quickly. Complications are few but if a woman has the disease during the first four months of pregnancy, she may have a deformed child.

Rugae. Wrinkles or creases.

Rugine. Instrument for elevating the periosteum.

Ropia. A skin disease with crusts due to tertiary syphilis.

Rupture, A bursting. In popular language a rupture means a hernia. In obstetric practice *rupture of the perineum* is not uncommon as a result of labour, especially in primiparae; *rupture of the uterus* is a rare event due to unrelieved obstructed labour, or more rarely still to unskillful attempts at delivery by the use of instruments; *rupture of the membranes* is the normal sequence of full dilatation of the cervix in labour, and marks the commencement of the second stage. *Rupture of a tubular extra-uterine pregnancy* may result in severe internal haemorrhage and would require immediate operation.

Resale traction. Method to reduce a fractured femur. There is an upward pull to a Balkan beam from a sling beneath the knee and from the lower part of the leg a longitudinal pull towards the foot of bed. The resultant direction of the pull helps to straighten the femur.

S

Sabin's vaccine. One of the poliomyelitis vaccines. It is taken orally.

Saccharin. An intensely sweet substance used as a substitute for sugar. It has no food value.

Saccharomyces. A group of fungi including yeasts. One is the cause of thrush.

Sacro-iliac synchondrosis or joint. The articulation between the sacrum and the hip bone. Normally there is no movement at this joint. During pregnancy the joint becomes more movable and this, to a slight extent, facilitates the birth of the child.

Sacrum. A wedge-shaped bone consisting of five fused vertebrae. They from the posterior wall of the pelvic cavity.

Sadism. A sexual perversion in which pleasure is derived from inflicting cruelty upon another.

Salicylate. A salt of salicylic acid, *e.g sodium salicylate* used in rheumatism. It relieves pain and reduces the temperature. *Methyl salicylate* (chief constituent of oil of winter green) is applied to painful joints.

Salicylic acid. An antiseptic used on the skin. *See* SALICYLATE. Acetyl-salicylic acid is aspirin.

Saline. Containing salt. *Physiological salin solution* is 0.91 per cent. This is isotonic with the blood. Sterile saline is given intravenously or subcutaneously.

Saliva. The secretion of the salivary glands.

Salivary glands, Three pairs of glands. The sublingual and submaxillary situated in the floor of the mouth; the parotid above the angle of the lower jaw. *See* PAROTID.

Salivation, The act of secretion of saliva.

Salk vaccine. One of the vaccines given to protect against poliomyelitis.It contains dead virus.

Selpingectomy. Remove of one or both Fallopian tubes.

Salpingocyesis. Tubal pregnancy.

Salpingography. Examination of the Fallopian tubes by x-rays.

Salpingo-oophorectomy. The surgical removal of Fallopian tubes and ovaries.

Salpingostomy. Opening artificially a Fallopian tube whose aperture has been closed by inflammation or previous surgery.

Salpinx. A tube, either Eustachina or Fallopian.

Sanatorium. Any institution for convalescent patients can techincally be called a sanatorium; but until recently indicated an institution for the open-air treatment of tuberculosis.

Sandfly fever. Tropical disease due to infection by organism transmitted by sandfly bites.

Samtation. The use of methods conducive to the public health.

Saphenous nerve, Large branch of the femoral nerve.

Saphenous opening. Just below groin near inner side of thigh where superficial saphenous vein passes deep to enter femoral vein.

Saphenous veins. Superficial leg veins. *Long s.v.* begins on the foot and extends to the groin. *Short s.v.* joins the popliteal vein at the knee.

Saprophytes. Organisms that exist only in dead matter.

Sarcoidosis. A systemic granulomatous disease of unknown cause, *i. e.* lesions being histologically similar to tuberculosis follicles. Affects lymph nodes, lungs, liver, spleen, skin, eyes, parotid glands and phalanges.

Sarcolemma. The membrane which covers each fibril of muscle.

Sarcology. Anatomy of the soft tissues as distinguished from osteology.

Sarcoma. A malignant tumour composed of embryonic connective tissue. Spread is by way of the blood-stream, and metastases are found in lungs, brain, and other organs.

Sartorius. The long ribbon-shaped muscle of the front of the thigh.

Scab. An incrustation formed over a wound.

Scabies. A contagious skin disease due to a parasitic insect, the acarus scabiei or Sarcoptes scabiei.

Scald. Burn caused by hot fluids.

Scale. The horny epidermis the skin sheds.

Scalp. The skin covering the cranium.

Scalpel. A straight knife with convex edge, used in dissecting and surgery.

Scaphoid. Boat-shaped. The name of a bone of the carpus and of the tarsus.

Scapula. The shoulder blade.

Scar. The connective fibrous tissue found after any wound has healed.

Scarification. Shallow incisions just penetrating the epidermis. A technique used in vaccination.

Scarlatina. Scarlet fever; an infectious fever. There is a widespread erythematous rash produced by a toxin released by haemolytic streptococci.

Scarpa's triangle. The femoral triangle bounded by Poupart's ligament, the adductor longus and sartorius.

SCAT. Sheep cell agglutination test. A serum test for rheumatoid arthritis.

Scheuermann's disease. Vertebral osteochondritis found in adolescents. It affects the two rings of cartilage and bone around the margin of both superior and inferior surfaces of the vertebral body. The condition does not cause general ill-health.

Schick test. A test for antibody in the patient's blood to the Klebs-Loeffler bacillus which causes diphtheria. A minute amount of diphtheria toxin (and protein) is injected into the patient's left forearm. If there is antitoxin in the patient's blood the toxin will be neutralized and there will be no reaction. If the patient's blood has little or no anti-toxin, there will be an area of redness on the skin 1 cm in diameter, within 24 hours, reaching its height in four days. This patient is susceptible to diphtheria. A control solution containing protein and inactive toxin is injected into the right arm. If there is a protein reaction or false reaction, this reaches its height in 24 hours and then fades.

Schizomycetes. A group of fungi which includes the yeasts.

Schizophrenia. Term used for a group of mental disorders characterized by a progressive loss of emotional stability, judgement and contact with reality.

Schlatter's disease. Osteochondritis of the anterior tubercle of the tibia. Also called Osgood-Schlatter's disease.

Schultz-Charlton reaction. Test to confirm scarlet fever. Antitoxin is injected into the skin where the rash is bright red. If the disease is present, there is a blanching ring round the injection site in about 18 hours.

Sciatica. Neuralgia of the sciatic nerve—the large nerve of the thigh. It may be caused by pressure on the nerves in the spinal canal or the pelvis.

Scissor-leg deformity. Deformity due to exaggerated tone in the adductor muscles usually resulting from cerebral damage.

Sclera. The opaque outer coat of the eyeball, forming five-sixths of the globe of the eye, the remaining one-sixth being formed by the cornea. *see* EYE.

Scleritis. An inflamed sclera.

Scleroderma. A collagen disease affecting the dermis causing contracture and deformities of joints and widespread systemic effects.

Scoliosis Lateral. Curvature of the spine.

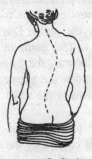

Scoliosis

Screening. Radiological examination by means of a fluorescent screen.

Scrofuloderma. Tuberculous condition of the skin.

Scrotocele. Hernia in the scrotum.

Scrotum. The bag which holds the testicles.

Acurf. Dandruff. Scales from the epidermis of the scalp.

Scurvy. A rare deficiency disease, due to an extremely low intake of vitamin C. *See* VITAMINS. Characterized by swelling of the gums, haemorrhages into skin and subcutaneous tissues, and from mucous membranes, and by anaemia. *Infantile s.* A type of the above occurring in infancy, characterized by subperiosteal haemorrhages and anaemia. Due to same cause.

Scybala. Faeces passed as hard dry masses.

Sebaceous. Fatty, secreting oily matter, *S. glands*, of skin, secrete fatty material called sebum. *S. cysts*, dilatation of one of these glands, due to blocking of its opening on to the skin. Cyst is filled with sebum.

Secondary areola. A peculiar pigmentation of the skin often seen on the breast around the nipple during pregnancy.

second stage. From complete dilatation of the cervix, usually associated with rupture of the membranes, to the complete expulsion of the child. During this stage, which lasts normally two to four hours in primigravidae, and up to one hour in multiparae, the pains are very severe, and the uterine contractions are assisted by those of the abdominal muscles. This is the stage for which anaesthetics are often given.

Secretin. A hormone formed in the mucous membrane of the duodenum. It is carried by the blood to the pancreas, exciting it to activity. It also stiumlates the secretion of bile.

Sedative. Drug allaying excitement or pain, *e.g.* morphia and barbiturates.

Sella turcica. Pituitary fossa of the sphenoid bone.

Semen. The secretion of the testicles mixed with that of the seminal vesicles and prostate.

Semicircular canals. Three canals of the internal ear, the sense organs of equilibrium or balance.

Semilunar cartilages. Menisci. Two crescentic cartilages, an internal and an external, lying in the knee joint between the femur and tibia. These may be torn and displaced. giving rise to pain and deformity and fluid in the knee joint. Usually removed by operation.

Seminal. Relating to the semen. *S. vesicles.* Two small structures in the male genito-urinary system which secrete part of the seminal fluid.

Senility. Degenerative changes due to advanced age.

Sensory nerves. Afferent nerves carrying sensory information to the central nervous system. Cf. motor nerves.

Sepsis. The condition of being infected by pyogenic bacteria.

Septicaemia. The circulation and multiplication of microorganisms in the blood; a very serious condition.

Septum. The division between two cavities; such as *septum ventriculorum*, which separates the right ventricle of the heart from the left.

Sequelae. Morbid conditions remaining after, and consequent on, some former illness.

Sequestrectomy. Operation to remove sequestrum.

Serotonin. Amine found in blood platelets, the intestines and brain substance. Mono-amine oxidase inactivates it.

Serum. (1) The fluid part of the blood, after clot and cells have been removed. (2) Fluid used for providing passive immunity against infection. The serum is taken from an animal which has been rendered immune against a certain pathogenic micro-organism, and which therefore must contain a large quantity of antibodies to that microorganism. The best known are the antidiphtheritic and the antitetanic sera. The antibodies contained in the injected serum combine chemically with the disease toxins, rendering the latter harmless. *S. sickness.* Late reaction to serum injections, arising eight to ten days after. *Symptoms*: Oedema, urticarial rash, joint pains, slight temperature.

Sesamoid bones. Small foci of bone formation in the tendons of muscles. The patella is the largest.

Sex. State of being male or female. *S. linked.* Characteristics not inherited equally by both sexes.

Sheehan's syndrome. Panhypopituitarism resulting from thrombosis of the pituitary blood supply occurring in association with post- partum haemorrhage.

Shiga's bacillus. The shigella dysenteriae. A cause of dysentery, especially in the Far East.

Shock. General depression of the vital functions. Most common after haemorrhage, severe injuries, or operations or in toxaemic states. The essential factor in shock is a deficiency in the volume of the blood in active circulation.

Short-sighted. Myopic.

Shoulder presentation. A form of transverse lie which must be converted into breech or vertex before delivery is possible.

Sialectasis. Dilatation of salivary gland due to obstruction to the flow of saliva.

Sialogogue. A medicine causing increased salivation, *e.g.* pilocarpine.

Sibilus. A hissing sound heard on auscultation of the chest during respiration in bronchitis, etc.

Sibling. One of two or more children of the same parents.

Sickle-cell anaemia. Hereditary anemia found sometimes in negroes. The red blood cells become sickle-shaped or crescentic.

Sigmoidoscope. An instrument for viewing the interior of the rectum and sigmoid flexure of the colon.

Sigmoidostomy. Opening into the sigmoid colon.

Silicosis. Lung disease due to the inhalation of the very fine particles of silica which irritate the lungs causing fibrotic changes.

Silkworm gut. A suture material much used by surgeons for sewing up abdominal wounds. It is very strong, not absorbed, and can be sterilized by boiling.

Silver nitrate. When solid this substance constitutes *lunar caustic*: used to destroy excess granulation tissue; it burns the skin and stains it dark brown or black. In weak solution it is used as an antiseptic.

Sims' position. The patient lies in the semi-prone position, across the bed. The buttocks are brought to the edge of the bed. The right knee is flexed more than the left. Used for vaginal examination.

Sinuatrial node. Cells found in the heart at the junction of the superior vena cava and the right atrium. The node is the pacemaker of the heart.

Sinus. (1) A passage leading from an abscess, or some inner part to an external opening. (2) A dilated channel for venous blood, *e.g. lateral s.*, large venous channel on inner side of the skull. It passes near the mastoid antrum and empties itself into the jugular vein (3) Air sinuses, hollow cavities in the skull bones which communicate with the nose. They are the frontal, maxillary, ethmoidal and sphenoidal sinuses.

Sinus arrhythmia. Irregular cardiac rhythm due to the controlling effect of the vagus on the sinuatrial node. The heart rate increases on inspiration and Nows during expiration.

Sinusitis. Inflammation of a sinus, especially one of the air sinuses of the bones of the skull.

Sjögren's syndrome. Keratoconjunctivities and dry mouth usually in postmenopausal women.

Skatole. A nitrogenous product of protein digestion found in the faeces.

Skeleton. The bony framework of the body (see illustration).

The skeleton

Labels: Skull, Vartebral column, Clavicle, Scapula, Sternum, Ribs, Humerus, Pelvis, Radius, Ulne, Carpals, Metacarpals, phalanges, Femur, patella, Tibia, Fibula, Tarsals, Metatrsals, Phalanges

Skene's glands. These open into posterior wall of the female urethra, just within the orifice; almost always infected in acute gonorrhoea.

Skin. The outer covering of the body consisting of epidermis and its appendages supported by specialized dermal connective tissue.

Skull. The bony framework of the head.

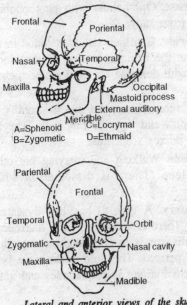

A=Sphenoid C=Locrymal
B=Zygometic D=Ethmaid

Lateral and anterior views of the skull

Sleeping sickness. Tropical disease due to a trypanosome. The tsetse fly carries the organisms which are transferred to healthy individuals by the bite of the fly.

Sleepy sickness. Encephalitis lethargica. A form of viral encephalitis.

Slough. Dead matter, thrown off by gangrene or ulcers.

Smallpox. A highly infectious disease caused by a virus. Incubation period 12-14 days. There is high temperature, headache, backache and cough, Rash appears on the fourth day and the temperature falls, but rises again and pustulation occurs and the patient becomes very ill.

Smith-Petersen nail. Inserted to fix the two fragments of bone in a fracture of the neck of the femur.

Snow blindness. Ophthalmia with photophobia caused by the glare from snow.

Sodium chloride. Common salt. It is found in the body and main- tains the osmotic tension of the blood. Given in infusions with dextrose for fluid replacement in dehydration.

Soft sore. A venereal sore not due to syphilis. Also known as chancroid, and *non-infecting* sore. The infecting organism is ducrey's bacillus.

Somnambulism. Walking and carrying out other activities whilst asleep. There is dissociation which may be hysterical.

Sonne dysentery. A type of bacillary dysentery. Common in Britain. There is abdominal pain, diarrhoea and vomiting. The disease is usually slight except in infants and debilitated persons. The fluid intake must be adequate to prevent dehydration. Sulphonamides and antibiotics may be used.

Soporific. An agent which induces sleep, *e.g.* chloral.

Sordes. Brown crusts about the lips and teeth of a feverish patient which should be removed during routine oral toilet.

Sound. A probe-like instrument used for exploring cavities such as the uterus, bladder, etc.

Southey's tubes. Small perforated metal tubes, used to

drain oedematous tissue.

Spasm. (1) Sudden convulsive involuntary movement. (2) Sudden contraction of a muscle or muscles, especially of the unstriped muscle coats of arteries, intestines, heart, bronchi, etc. The effect of such spasm depends on the part affected: thus asthma is believed to be due to spasm of the muscular coats of the smaller bronchi; and renal colic is due to spasm of the muscle coat of the ureter.

Spasticity. The condition of being spastic. Occurs in an upper motor neurone lesion.

Spatula. (1) A flat, flexible, blunt knife, used for spreading ointments and poultices. (2) A tongue depressor.

Speculum. A polished instrument for polished instrument for examining the interior cavities of the body, especially the vagina, the rectum, the ear, and the nose.

Speech center. The parts of the brain controlling speech.

Speech therapist. One trained to treat defects and disorders of language, voice and speech.

Spencer-Wells forceps. The usual forceps for heemostasis during operations.

Sperm. Semen.

Spermatic cord. Composed of arteries, veins. lymphatics and nerves, and the vas deferens (the duct of the testicle); it suspends the testicle from the abdomen.

Spermatocele. A retention cyst from some part of the epididymis.

Spermatozoa. The male generative cells; minute cells found in the semen, which are possessed of the power of self-propulsion by means of a flagellum, and which can fertilize the ovum, or female germ cell.

Spermicide. Substance destroying spermatozoa.

Sphenoid. Wedge-shaped. The name of one of the bones forming the base of the skull.

Sphygmocardiograph. Apparatus recording both pulse and heart, beats.

Sphygmograph. An instrument affixed to the wrist, which moves with the beat of the pulse and registers the rate and character of the beats.

Sphygmomanometer. An instrument for measuring the arterial tension (or blood pressure) of the circulation.

Spina bifida. A congenital malformation of the spine due to the neural arch of one or more vertebrae failing to fuse in the mondline. The vertebral and is exposed at this site and may herniate through the opening. The defect most commonly occurs in the lumbo-sacral region.

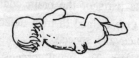

Spina bifida-meningocele

Spinal column. The backbone. It is composed of seven cervical, twelve thoracic and five lumbar vertebrae and the sacrum with its five fused vertebrae and the coccyx or tailbone.

Spinal cord. The portion of the central nervous system within the spine. It is composed of nerve cells and bundles of nerve fibres connecting the various levels of the spinal cord with the brain. Thirty-one pairs of spinal nerves form the peripheral nervous system of the trunk and limbs.

Spinal curvature. The *normal* curvature of the spine is divided into primary curvature giving an open like stooping porture and secondary curvatures (cervical and lumbar). For abnormal spinal curvature *see* SCOLIOSIS, KYPHOSIS, LORDOSIS.

Spine. The backbone or spinal column.

Spirochaetaemia. The presence of spirochaetes in the blood.

Spirograph. Instrument for recording respirations.

Spirometer. An instrument for measuring the capacity of the lungs.

Splanchnicectomy. Surgical removal of the splanchnic ganglia and transaction of the splanchnic nerves.

Spleen. A mass of lymphoid tissue situated in the mesentery of the abdomen. Unlike the lymph nodes, the spleen acts as a filtration organ for blood. The spleen forms an important part of the reticulo-endothelial system, and is the generative center of the formation of many lymphocytes. The spleen is largely responsible for the removal of red blood cells at the end of their lifespan.

Splenectomy. Removal of the spleen.

Splints. Used to immobilize a limb in the case of fracture, disease or deformity. They are now made chiefly or plaster of paris, metal, rarely of wood, and the limb is slung on pieces of material attached to sides of splints. The aim is to immobilize the limb as required, at the same time allowing as much movement as possible.

Spondyle. A vertebra.

Spondylitis. Inflammation of a vertebra or vertebrae. *Ankylosing s.* Condition of unknown origin occurring characteristically in young men. There is ossification of spinal ligaments with ankylosis of the cervical and sacro-iliac joints.

Spondylolisthesis. The vertebral arch of the fifth lumbar vertebra gives way so that the body of the affected vertebra becomes displaced.

Spondylosis. Degenerative changes in the intervertebral discs with peripheral ossification. Known as 'osteo-arthritis of spines'.

Spontaneous fracture. Fracture due to disease affecting the bone, either from abnormal development or rarefaction of the bone from other cause.

Spotted fever. Cerebrospinal meningitis.

Sprain. Severe strain of a joint without fracture or disloca-tion, but with swelling and often with effusion into joint.

Sputum. Expectorated matter. Different types are: *Mucoid*, occurs in the early stage of irritation. *Muco-purulent* develops at a later stage, pus is mixed with mucus. *Rusty*, tenacious sputum occurs in lobar pneumonia. Copious foul smelling sputum occurs in bronchiectasis. Forthy sputum occurs in oedema of the lung. Separate pellets or nummular sputum occurs in pulmonary tuber-culosis. It may be streaked with blood.

Stacke's operation. Operation used in chronic infection to join the middle ear with that of the mastoid cells.

Staphylococcus. Genus of Gram-positive bacteria which grow in clusters when cultured. Many staphylococci are commensals on the skin. Some are serious pathogens and several strains have evolved which are insensitive to penicillin and other antibiotics.

Staphyloma. Any protrusion of the sclerotic or corneal

coats of the eyeball due to inflammation.

Stasis. Standing still. Most commonly used for arrest of the circulation of either blood or lymph, but also for intestinal stasis, a holding up of the contents of the bowel.

Status asthmaticus. Severe attack of asthma unrelieved by usual medication.

Status epilepticus. A condition in which a series of epileptic fits occur in rapid succession.

Status lymphaticus. A rare and fatal condition in which death in sudden and thought in some case to be due to persistent thymus gland.

Stegomyia. A variety of mosquito which acts as the carrier of the parasite of yellow fever from a patient to a healthy individual.

Stein-Leventhal syndrome. Sterility, uterine hypoplasia, masculinization and polycystic ovaries.

Steinmann's pin. A fixation pin inserted through a bone in order to apply extension in the case of fractures.

Stensen's duct. The duct of the parotid salivary gland. Its opening is opposite the upper first molar tooth.

Stercobilin. The colouring matter of the faeces. It is derived from bile pigment.

Stercolith. Small hard mass of faeces. Faecolith.

Stereognosis. Recognition of the form of bodies by handing them.

Sterile. Barren; unable to have children. In *surgical* practice, sterile means entirely free from microorganisms of all kinds, a result brought about by heat or by the use of chemicals.

Sterility. The condition of being sterile.

Sterilization. (1) Made incapable of progeny, *e.g.* by

removal of ovaries, tying the Fallopian tubes, hysterectomy or, in the male, castration, tying the vas deferens. (2) Rendering free of micro-organisms.

Sternal puncture. Technique employed to obtain simple of red bone marrow for investigation. A needle is inserted into the sternum under local anesthesia and a small amount of marrow aspirated.

Sternum. The breastbone.

Steroids. Group of compounds including cholesterol, most of the hormones, bile salts and the precursors of vitamin D in the skin. However, the term is often used for the corticosteroids only, which are the hormones of the adrenal cortex.

Stertor. Snoring type of respiration.

Stethoscope. Instrument for listening to sounds, *e.g.* heart sounds, respiratory sounds. The *binaural* stethoscope has two flexible ends, to apply to the ears of the listener.

Stevens-Johnson syndrome. Severe form of erythema multiforme in which mucous membranes may be extensively involved.

Stigma. Mark of the skin.

Stillborn. Dead when born.

Still's disease. Refers to a form of rheumatoid arthritis occurring in children. The syndrome is characterized by polyarthritis, lymph adenopathy, splenomegaly, calcification of the cornea and formation of cataract.

Stimulant. That which causes temporary increase in the output of the vital energy.

Stitch. (1) Suture. (2) Pain in the side due to spasm of the diaphragm.

Stokes-Adams' syndrome. Syncope due to cerebral hypoxia

resulting from heart block.

Stoma. (1) The mouth. (2) An opening onto the skin, e.g. colostomy; *s. nurse* one who undergoes further training in care of patients with stomas.

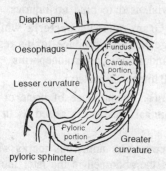

Diaphragm
Oesophagus
Fundus
Cardiac portion
Lesser curvature
Pyloric portion
Greater curvature
pyloric sphincter

Section through the stomach

Stomach. Refers to the dilated portion of the intestinal canal into which the food passes from the esophagus, and where it undergoes partial digestion.

Stomach pump. A thick rubber tube, at least 18 inches long, attached to a glass receptacle which has a rubber bulb inserted into its neck by means of which a vacuum is created in the glass flask. Used to aspirate the contents of the stomach.

Stomatitis. Inflammation of the mouth.

Stone. (1) A measure of weight, 14 pounds. (2) A concretion.

Stools. Discharge of faces from the bowels.

Strabismus. Squint; divergent when the eye turns out; *convergent* when it turns in.

Strabotomy. Operation to remedy squinting.

Strangulated. Constricted, so that the blood-supply is cut off.

Strangury. Painful passage of urine. Usually the result of disease of the bladder, urethra, broad ligament, etc. but occasionally occurs after labour.

Strapping. Material used to bind up injuries.

Streptococcus. Gram-positive bacteria which grow in chains. Pathogenic cocci produce toxins responsible for scarlet fever and acute glomerulonephritis.

Streptothrix. Fillamentous bacteria.

Stress incontinence. Incontinence of urine or fasces when the intra-abdominal pressure is raised as in coughing or sneezing.

Striaeg gravidarum. The numerous marks which develop on the skin of the abdomen in the later months of pregnancy. They never quite disappear. Striae are due to the stretching of the skin, and are seen also in any condition of rapid enlargement of the abdomen, and also sometimes on the thighs of boys who are growing very rapidly. They are thought to be associated with increased activity of the suprarenal cortex.

Striated muscle. Striped voluntary muscle, *cf. smooth muscle.*

Stricture. Contraction. Usually applied to the urethra, with consequent inability to pass urine.

Stridor. A harsh sound during breathing, caused by obstruction to the passage of air.

Stroke. Cerebrovascular accident.

Stroma. The connective tissue.

Stupe, A fomentation sprinkled with a counterirritant, *e.g.* turpentine.

Stupor. State of unconsciousness.

Sturge-Weber syndrome. Syndrome characterized by capillary naevus on the face in the distribution of the fifth cranial nerve. Associated with angiomas of the cerebral cortex which may cause focal epilepsy, hemiparesis and mental deficiency.

Stye. Hordeolum. Inflammation of sebaceous gland of eyelash.

Styptic. Agent applied to arrest bleeding; astringent, *e.g.* adrenalin.

Stypven. Local aemostatic containing Rusell's viper venom.

Subacute bacterial endocarditis. Bacterial colonization of defective heart valves with consequent bacteraemia and distribution of septic emboli throughout the body.

Subacute combined degeneration of the cord. Degeneration of the posterior and lateral columns of the spinal cord due to vitamin B^2 deficiency.

Subarachnoid haemorrhage. Haemorrhage into the subarachnoid space.

Subarachnoid space, The space between the arachnoid membrane and the piarmatter. It contains cerebrospinal fluid.

Subclavian. Under the clavicle: thus the subclavian artery and vein are vessels passing under the clavicle.

Subclinical. Without any obvious signs of the disease.

Subconscious. The part of the mind outside an individual's awareness, but able to affect the way of acting or thinking.

Subcutaneous. Under the skin.

Subinvolution. Failure of the lately pregnant uterus to regain the normal unimpregnated size within the usual time (six weeks) of delivery.

Succus entericus. The digestive juice secreted by the glands in the small intestine.

Succession. Sound made on shaking a patient if fluid is present in a hollow cavity.

Sudamina. Sweat rash.

Sudol. A phenol preparation having the same wide range of bactericidal power as Lysol, but with reduced neurotic action on the skin.

Sudorific. An agent causing perspiration.

Suffused. Congested.

Suggestibility. A state when the patient readily accepts other people's ideas and influences.

Suicide. The person who kills himself by intent.

Sulcus. A furrow.

Superciliary. Having to do with the eyebrows.

Supercilium. The eyebrow.

Superfecundation. The fertiliastion of two ova discharged by two distinct acts of insemination effected at a short interval.

Supplemental air. Refers to that part of the residual air of the lung which after the tidal air has been expelled may be driven out by forced respiration.

Suppository. Rectally administered cones containing a medicament in a base which is soluble at body temperature.

Suppuration. The formation of pus.

Sural. Relating to the calf of the leg.

Surgery. The part of medicine concerned with diseases needing treatment by operation. A physician or surgeon's consulting room.

Suspensory bandage. A bandage to support the testicle.

Sutures. (1) Silk, thread, catgut, nylon, etc., used to sew a wound. (2) The union of flat bones by their margins, *e.g.* bones of the skull.

Swabs. Small pieces of wool, gauze over wool, or gauze only, used for cleaning wounds and for removing blood at operations.

Sweat. Perspiration. The fluid secreted on to the skin by the sweat glands.

Sycosis. Inflammation of the hair follicles, especially of the beard and whiskers.

Symbiosis. The living together of two organisms, whose mutual association is necessary to each, although neither is parasitic on the other.

Symblepharon. Adhesion of the eyelids to the eyeball.

Syme's amputation. Amputation at the ankle joint.

Sympathectomy. Surgical transection of sympathetic nerves usually with excision of part of the sympathetic chain.

Sympathetic system, A nerve system consisting of a chain of ganglia beside the spine supplying nerves to the heart, bloodvessels and other internal viscera.

Symphysiotomy. The operation of dividing the symphysis pubis (of the mother) so as to facilitate delivery in certain cases of contracted pelvis.

Symphysis. Growing of bones together. The *symphysis pubis* is the bony mass bounding the front of the pelvis, at the lower end of the abdomen. *See* PELVIS.

Symptom. A noticeable change in the body and its functions, evidence of disease. Usually meaning the change complained of by the patient.

Symptomatology. A study of the symptoms of disease.

Synapse. Region where nerve cells communicate. There is

no continuity between the neurons and impulses are transmitted from one nerve cell to another by the passage of chemical messengers which stimulate the post-synaptic nerve cell.

Synarthrosis. Immovable union of bones, e.g. the cranial bones.

Synchondrosis. Joint whose surfaces are united by cartilage.

Synchysis. Softening of the vitreous humour of the eye. *S. Scintillans.* Bright particles found in the vitreous humour.

Synclitism. Descent of the fetal head through the pelvis with its planes parallel to those of the pelvis.

Syncope. Fainting.

Syndactyly. Webbed fingers or toes.

Syndesmitis. Inflammation of ligaments.

Syndrome. Refers to The collection of symptoms and signs which form a recognizable pattern of disease.

Synechia. Adhesion of the iris to the cornea, or to the crystalline lens.

Synergy. The working together of two or more agents.

Synkavit. A vitamin K analogue.

Synostosis. Means abnormal osseous union of bones.

Synovectomy. Operation to remove synovial membrane.

Synovial fluid. Refers to the liquid which lubricates the joints.

Synovial membrane. Refers to that lining a joint cavity but not covering the articular surfaces.

Synovitis. Inflammation of the synovial membrane of a joint.

Syphilide. Refers to the lesion of the skin due to syphilis. May be papular, macular, squamous, etc.

Syphilis. A venereal disease. Caused by a specific spirochaete, the Treponema pallidum. S. may be congenital or acquired. *Congenital* may be inherited from the mother. The chief symptoms in young babies: wasting, snuffles, rashes, enlargement of liver and spleen. If child survies, he may later show pallor, malnutrition, depressed bridge of nose, rhagades, square skull, thickening of tibiae, corneal opacities, Hutchinson's teeth. *Acquired* is divided into three stages. (1) First stage or primary S. with local symptoms, tow-three weeks after infection. Hard chancre on penis, vulva, or cervix. Inflamed glands in groin. Lesions infective (2) Second stage or secondary S., one to two months after infection, with rashes, sore throat, mucous patches, condylomata, general enlargement of glands, anaemia, and fever. Infective (3) Third stage or tertiary S., two to ten years or even longer after infection. Non-infective, giving, among other manifestations, gum mata, tabes, GPI.

Syringe. An instrument for injecting fluids, or for exploring and aspirating cavities.

Syringomyelia, Progressive degenerative disease affecting the brain stem and spinal cord in which the tract of the fibres subserving pain and temperature are mainly affected.

Syringomyelocele, Refers to a type of spina bifida. There is a communication between the projecting mass and the central canal of the spinal cord.

Syringotomy. Cutting open a fistula.

Systemic. Affecting the whole body.

Systole. The period when the heart contracts.

Systolic blood pressure. The force with which the left ventricle contracts and which is measured in the peripheral arteries.

Systolic murmur. Murmur heard during systole. It may be due to aortic or tricuspid obstruction.

TAB. Triple vaccine to prevent typhoid, paratyphoid. A and paratyphoid B.

T bandage. A special bandage used for keeping dressings on the perineum.

Tabes. Wasting. *T. dorsalis*, a disorder of the spinal cord, due to tertiary syphilis, also called locomotor ataxia, and characterized by loss of power over muscles. *See* SYPHILEIS. *T. mesenterica*, tuberculosis of the mesenteric glands. Seen in children.

Tachycardia. Abnormally rapid action of the heart, as in

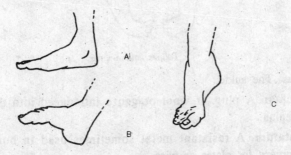

Types of talipes: A = talipes valgus B = talipes calcaneus with some cavus deformity C = talipes equinus.

atrial fibrillation.

Tactile. Relating to the touch.

Taenia. The tapeworm. The adult worm consists of a head and numerous segments. It has the appearance of jointed tape and may be several feet long. the *taenia solium* is a common variety which gains entrance to the body through underdone infected pork. The head attaches itself to the mucous membrane of the intestines and the worm continues to grow. The treatment is (1) little food for several hours, (2) purge, (3) ext. filix mas, (4) Purge.

Talc. French chalk. Used as dusting powdr.

Talipes. Clubfoot. *Talipes valgus*, the foot turned outwards; *varus*, the foot turned inwards; *equinus*, the heel lifted from the ground; *calcaneus*, heel projected downwards.

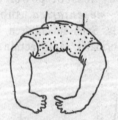

Talipes equino-varus

Talus. The ankle.

Tampon. A plug of wool or gauze introduced into the vagina.

Tantalum. A resistant metal sometimes used in bone surgery for plates or wire.

Tar. Dark liquid obtained from pine-wood. It has antiseptic properties. *Coal-t.* Black liquid distilled from coal. It contains benzene, phenol, cresols, naphthalene, etc.

Tarsal. Bones of the ankle. *cf.* carpal bones. There are seven in man, forming a group which articulate with the tibia and fibula and the metatarsal bones.

Tarsalgia. Pain in the foot.

Tarsoplasty. Plastic surgery of the eyelid.

Tarsorrhaphy. Stitching the eyelides together.

Tarsus. (1) The seven small bones of the foot. (2) The cartilaginous framework of the eyelid.

Tartar. Deposit on teeth of calcium salts derived from saliva.

Tartaric acid. Used in making effervescent preparations. It should be taken well-diluted if not neutralized.

Taste bud. Specialized sensory end organ which is sensitive to taste.

Taurocholic acid. One of the bile acids.

Taris. Hand-manipulation for restoring a part to its natural position, such as reducing a hernia.

Tay-Sach's disease. A rare genetically. inhesited neurological condition which also produces mental regression.

Tears. Secretion of the lacrimal gland.

Tease. To divide a tissue into shreds.

Teat. Nipple.

Teeth, eruption of. The milk teeth, or first dentition of the infant, begin to erupt between the sixth and twelfth months. Occasionally they start to appear even earlier than the sixth month. The lower central incisors usually appear first, followed by the upper central incisors. As a rule thre will be from eight to twelve teeth cut at a year old, and the twenty teeth which constitute the first dentition should be present at two years of age. The per-

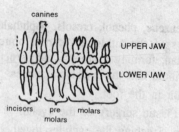

First dentition or temporary teeth

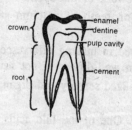

Second dentition or permanent teeth

manent teeth begin to erupt about the fifth or sixth year with the appearance of the first permanent molars; then about the seventh year there is shedding of the incisors. The numbers in the top illustration indicate the child's age in months when the teeth erupt.

Teflon. Proprietary material used in heart surgery.

Tegument. The skin.

Telangiectasis, telangioma. Lesion consisting a number of tortuous dilated capillaries which have a weblike appearance and a tendencey to bleed. Often seen following a course of radiotherapy.

Temper tantrums. Outburst of temper. An infantile way of demanding that a need be satisfied.

Temperament. A person's mental outlook.

Temperature. A measurement of the degree of heat. The average normal temperature of the human body is 98.6° F (37°C). The average temperature of a sick-room should be 60° to 65° F (16 to 18°C).

Temples. The part of the forehead between the outer corner of the eye and the hair.

Temporal. Relating to the temple. Thus T. artery, T. bone, T. lobe of the brain.

Temporal arteritis. A disease of unknown aetiology characterized by general malaise aches and muscle pains and acute inflammation of the arteries, particularly those of the scalp.

Tenaculum. An instrument like a vulsellum, but having only one pair of teeth for fixing the cervix uteri.

Tendinitis. Inflammation of a tendon.

Tendo Achilles. The stout tendon of the calf muscles at the back of the heel.

Tendon. A sinew, a cord of fibrous white tissue by which a muscle is attached to a bone or other structure.

Tendovaginitis, stenosing. Stenosing tenosynovitis, de Quervain's disease. Fibrous thickening of tendon sheath most commonly affecting the tendons of the abductor muscles of the thumb.

Tenesmus. Continual desire to defaecate accompanied by painful straining.

Tennis elbow. A condition characterized by pain at or near the insertion of the extensor muscles of the forearm at the lateral epicondyle of the humerus. Brought on by unusual and excessvie use.

Tenoplasty. Plastic surgery to a tendon.

Tenorrhaphy. Operation to suture a tendon.

Tenosynovitis. Inflammation in the sheath of a tendon.

Tenotomy. Cutting a tendon.

Tentorium cerebelli. A septum of the dura mate which lies between the cerebrum and cerebellum. This may be torn in a breech delivery and may prove fatal to the child.

Tepid spongig. A method of bringing down high temperature by allowing tepid water to evaporate on the skin. During the treament the patient must be watched carefully for signs of collapse and the temperature must not be allowed to drop by more than 1°C.

Teratogen Any agent able to produce a fetal monster.

Tertian. A form of malaria with attacks every third day.

Testicies. The two glands of the scrotum which secrete the semen.

Testis. A testicle.

Testosterone. Endocrine secretion of the testis. Promotes growth and secondary sexual development.

Tetanus. Lock-jaw. Disease caused by *clostridium tetani* characterized by rigidity and spasm of the mucles. The causative organism is anaerobic and thrives in wounds contaminated by soil or road dust containing the spores. A powerful toxin is produced by the clostridium which reaches the spinal cord by retrograde spread up the motor nerves, and is responsible for the clinical features.

Tetany. Refers to a condition marked by spasms of the exrtemities, particularly of hands and feet (carpopedal spasm) due to faulty calcium metabolism. It may be due to dysfunction of the parathyroid glands, alkalosis, rickets.

Tetralogy of Fallot. Congenital heart disease. The aorta is displaced to the right so that it receives blood from the right ventricle, which is hypertrophied, as well as from the left ventricle. The interventricular septum is patent and there is narrowing of the pulmonary artery.

Tetraplegia. Paralysis of all four limbs. Syn. quadriplegia.

Thalami. Two areas of grey matter at the base of the brain; concerned with the appreciation of crude sensations.

Thalassaemia. Anaemia found in the Mediterranean area. The red cells contain some abnormal haemoglobin of the type usually found in the fetus. It is detected by the alkali resistance test.

Theca. A sheath. Examples are the meninges of the spinal cord, and the synovial sheaths of the flexor tendons of the fingers.

Therapeutics. The branch of medicine which deals with treatment.

Thermography. A means of recording infra-red radiation from the body by the use of special cameras. A 'hot spot' suggests a malignant tumour.

Thermometer. An instrument used to measure temperature. *Clinical thermometer*, a small thermometer used for taking the temperature of the body. It is generally graduated from 36° C to 42° C. It is made so that the mercury does not fall when the thermometer is taken from the patient. After the temperature has been recorded the mercury is shaken down.

Thermostat. Apparatus which is made to regulate heat automatically.

Thesis. Dissertation.

Thiamine. Synthetic vitamin B^1. Also called aneurine.

Thiersch. Type of skin graft in which the epidermis and upper part of the dermis is employed.

Thigh. The portion of the lower limb above the knee.

Thomas's splint. (1) Knee splint for immobilizing a fractured femur or tibia and fibula. It consists of two sidepieces of metal with a crosspiece at foot, and an oblique ring for fixation in groin. Leg is kept in position by pieces of material slung between sidepieces and adjusted to the fracture. (2) Arm splint.

Thoracic duct. The largest lympathic vesssel. It receives the fat absorbed from the intestine and the lymp from the greater part of the body. It ascends from the abdomen through the thorax to the left side of the neck, where it empties itself into the angle of union between the left internal jugular vein and the subclavian vein.

Thoracocentesis. Puncture of the thorax, e.g. aspiration of the pleural effusion.

Thoracolysis. The severing of adhesions between the two layers of the pleura.

Thoracoscopy. The pleural cavity is inspected by a thoracoscope.

Thoracotomy. Operation of opening the thorax.

Thorax. The chest; the cavity which holds the heart and lungs.

Threadworm. Oxyuris vermicularis. Small parasitic worm in the rectum; common in children.

Threonine. An amino-acid essential for protein metabolism.

Thrill. A vibratory impulse perceived by palpation.

Thrombectomy. Removal of a blood clot.

Thrombin. Enzyme necessary for the clotting of shed blood. It causes fibrinogen to become fibrin.

Thromboangiitis. Inflamed blood vessel with formation of a blood clot. *T. obliterans.* Inflammatory, obliterative disease of the blood vessels, especially in the limbs.

Thrombo-arteritis. Arteritis with thrombosis.

Thrombocytes. Blood platelets.

Thrombocytopenia. Deficiency of platelets in the blood.

Thromboendarterectomy. Operation to remove a clot from a blood vessel.

Thrombokinase. The active principle of a substance liberated when the blood platelets ar disintegrated. It is necessary for the clotting of blood.

Thrombolytic. Causing a clot to disintegrate.

Thrombophlebitis. Inflammation of a vein with thrombosis.

Thrombosis. Coagulation of blood in the vessels. The organized clot thus formed is termed a *thrombus.*

Thrombus. A clot of blood found in the heart or in a blood vessel in the site in which it is formed, *cf.* infarct.

Thymectomy. Operation to remove the thymus gland. Sometimes performed for myasthenia gravis.

Thymol. An antiseptic often used for mouthwashes and gargles.

Thymoma. Malignant neoplasm of the thymus.

Thymus. A gland at the root of the neck. It is largest in children and then gradually atrophies. The function of the thymus is not clear. It appears to be concerned with the immunological mechanisms of the body. It has been suggested that it acts as a 'priming station' for lymphocytes where they are selected for release into the general circulation. It is not yet possible to be certain of its function. The gland, which is situated in the anterior mediastinum, reaches its maximum size at puberty and thereafter atrophies slowly.

Thyroglossal cyst. A type of dermoid cyst which appears in the midline of neck between hyoid bone and sternum.

Thyroid cartilage. The largest cartilage of the larynx. It forms an angle in front, more prominent in the male.

Thyroid crisis. Actue severe thyrotoxicosis which may follow subtotal thyroidectomy in the absence of preoperative antithyroid treatment. Rarely occurs nowadays because of preoperative medication.

Thyroidectomy. Operative removal of the thyroid gland.

Thyroid gland. A bi-lobed ductless gland lying in front of the trachea. It secretes two thyroid hormones, thyroxine and triiodothyronine. These control metabolism, growth the development. Congenital lack causes cretinism. Unersecretion in later life causes myxoedema. Excessive secretion causes thyrotoxicosis. A third hormone, calcitonin, plays a part in calcium metabolism.

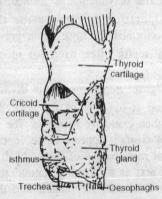

The thyroid gland

Thyroeidism. Refers to the symptoms caused by too rapid an absorption into the system of the secretion of the thyroid gland or by the administration by mouth of too large doses of thyroid extract, *Symptoms*: rapid pulse, sweating diarrhoea weight loss in spite of increased appetite, prominence of the eyeballs, fine tremor of the fingers and anxiety.

Thyrotoxicosis, Condition produced by over-activity of thyroid gland.

Thyroxine. One of the thyroid hormones Known as T4 because its molecule contains 4 iodine atoms.

Tibia. The shin bone the larger bone of the leg below the knee. *See* SKELETION.

Tic. Spasmodic twitching of muscles; usually of face and neck.

Tick. A blood sucking parasite. *T. fever* (1) relapsing fever. (2) Rocky Mountain fever, a rickettsial fever.

Tidal air. That which is inspired and expired during normal breathing.

Tincture. An alcoholic solution of a drug.

Tinea. Disease of the skin due to a vegetable parasite. *See* RINGWORM.

Tinnitus aurium. A ringing in the ears.

Tissue. the arrangement of cells constituting the structure of an organ.

Tissue culture. Method by which cells and tissues are grown under artificial conditions after their removal from the parent organism.

Tobacco amblyopia. Dimness of vision from excessive smoking.

Tocography. Method of recording alteration in the intrauterine pressure.

Tocopheryl. Vitamin E. Its precise function is unknown but it is widely used as antioxidant in medical preparation.

Tolerance, Capacity to take a certain drug in unusually large dosage.

Tomogrphy. The technique in radiography which brings into focus only those objects lying in the plane of interest while blurring structures on either side of the object's plane; also known as body section radiography.

Tone. (1) State of tension as found in muscles. (2) Quality of sound.

Tongue. The muscular organ which lies in thee floor of the mouth, and whose chief functions are to assist in the mastication and tasting of food and in vocalization.

Tongue tie. When a fold of mucous membrane attaches the under surface of tongue to floor of mouth. It is very rare.

Tonic. (1) A medicine which braces up the general health chiefly by increasing the appetite. (2) Term applied to continuous spasms, in opposition to clonic.

Tonometer. Instrument for measuring tensions such as that used to measure intra-ocular tension.

Tonsillectomy. the operation for removal of the tonsils.

Tonsillitis. Inflammation of tonsils.

Tonsillotome. An instrument for cutting off a tonsil.

Tonsils. Two oval bodies of lymphoid tissue on either side of the throat at the opening of the pharynx and between the pillars of fauces.

Toothed. Dentate. Possessing teeth.

Topical. Pertaining to a particular locality. local.

Topography. A study of the various areas of the body.

Torpor. Lethargy.

Torsion. Twisting.

Torso. The trunk.

Torticollis. Wryneck. The head is flexed and drawn to one side due to damage to one of the sternomastoid muscles at birth.

Tourniquet, An instrument which is used to exert pressure on an artery and so arrest bleeding.

Toxaemia, Circulation of toxins in the blood *Toxaemia of pregnancy.* The chief signs and symptoms are oedema, rise in blood pressure, proteinuria, headache and vomiting. If not treated, eclampsia may result.

Toxic. Poisonous.

Toxicology. Science of poisons.

Toxicosis. Any disease due to poisoning.

Toxin. A poison, usually of bacterial origin, *i.e.* manufactured by the germs themselves.

Toxoid. A non-poisonous modification of a toxin. Sometimes used to immunize against disease.

Toxoid-antitoxin. A mixture of toxoid and its antitoxin.

Toxoplasmosis. Infection caused by a parasite, the Toxoplasma, which can infect man as well as animals. If the fetus or young infant is infected encephalitis may occur. Other results of infection include nephritis pneumonia, rashes and lymphadenopathy.

Trabecula. A septum extending into an organ from its capsule or wall.

Trace elements. Mineral substances whose presence in minute amounts in the diet is necessary for the maintenance of health, *e.g* cobalt, copper, manganese, etc.

Tracer. Radioactive isotope or substance containing a radioactive isotope which enables the substance to be raced in metabolic systems.

Trachea. The wind-pipe; the air passage from the larynx to the bronchi.

Tracheitis. Inflammation of the trachea.

Trachelorrhaphy. The operation of suturing a torn cervix uteri.

Tracheobronchitis. Inflammation of trachea and bronchi.

Tracheostomy. The operation of making an opening into the trachea and inserting a tube. This may be performed in cases of respiratory obstruction and in cases where the patient is to be maintained on a ventilator.

Trachoma. A contagious disease of the conjunctiva in which eyelids become red, rough and granular and the cornea becomes opaque.

Traction. The act of pulling or dragging. *Skeletal.* Traction on a long bone to keep it in position after a fracture and to prevent muscle spasm.

Tragus. The small eminence just inside the ear.

Trait. A special characteristic of the individual.

Tranquillizer. Drug with sedative and tranquillizing action, such as chlorpromazine. Used to relieve anxiety, tension and agitation in psychotherapy. Whilst the patient is taking this drug, the action of a hypnotic or analgesic is made more powerful.

Transillumination. The method where by suppuration in the maxillary or frontal sinus is detected. The patient is placed in a completely darkened room, and a bright light placed in the mouth. The affected side is not so highly illuminated as the sound side.

Transmigration. The passage of cells through a membrane remove a portion of tissue from one part of the body to another.

Transposition of vessels. Defect of development in which the pulmonary artery arises from the left ventricle and the aorta from the right ventricle.

Transudation. Oozing of fluid through a membrane or from a tissue.

Trapezium. First bone in second row of carpal bones.

Trapezius. A large muscle, running from the nape of the neck and the upper part of the spine, to the clavicle and scapula.

Traperzoid. Second bone in second row of carpal bones.

Trauma. A wound or injury. Thus *traumatic gangrene* is gangrene arising from an injury.

Treatment. A way of curing a disease. *Conservative t.* Treatment by rest and drugs rather than by surgery. In dentistry, treatment of tooth without extracting it. *Palliative t.* An attempt to alleviate pain, etc., but not a cure for the disease. *Prophylactic t.* A means of preventing the disease such as by immunization against it, or by avoiding the cause.

Trematoda. Parasites which infect man, causing bilharzia.

Tremor. Involuntary trembling.

Trendelenburg's operation. Used to treat varicose veins. The long saphenous vein is ligated in the groin.

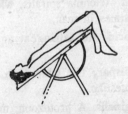

The Trendelenburg position

Trendelenburg position. A position often adopted for patients undergoing gynaecological operations, in which the head is at a lower level than the pelvis, and the latter is lower than the knees.

Trandelenburg's sign. Used to diagnose congenital dislocation of hip, etc. if the abductor muscles are not working properly, when the patient stands only on the affected leg, the pelvis tilts down wards on the opposite side.

Trephine. An instrument for removeving a disc of bone. *Elliot's t.* for removing a minute disc from the eyeball to relieve glaucoma.

Trephining. Removing a circular piece of tissue to gain access to an enclosed structure, *e.g* trephining the bone of the skull.

Treponema pallidum. The infecting agent of syphilis.

Trial of labour. Attempt to achieve spontaneous delivery in case of disproprotion.

Triangular bandage. Made by cutting a 36 inch square of linen diagon ally across. It is very useful in emergencies and for minor casualties.

Triceps. Certain muscles with three heads especially the one at the back of the arm which extends the elbow.

Trichiasis. Inversion of the eyelashes towards the eye.

Trichiniasis, trichinosis. Infection with a parasitic worm named *Trichina.* Trichina spiralis, which is parasitic in pigs and sometimes in man.

Trichloroacetic acid. An astringent and caustic used to remove warts.

Trichocephalus dispar. The whipworm. A parasite of the human large intestine.

Trichomonas vaginalis. A protozoon, motile by means of flagellae. It is a common cause of non-venereal vaginitis.

Trichonosis trichopathy. Any disease of the hair.

Trichophytosis. Fungus infection of the hair caused by trichophyton.

Tricuspid valve. Valve with three cusps, particularly the valve of the heart between the right atrium and right ventricle.

Trigeminal nerves. Fifth pair of cranial nerves. They are motor an sensory and each has three branches supplying the skin and structures of the face tongue and teeth.

Trigeminal neuralgia. Pain in the face of unknown cause. The distribution is confined to branches of the trigeminal .nerve. The pain is paroxysmal and precipitated by mild stimuli such as washing the f`ce or eating. Syn. tic douloureux.

Trigger finger. A thickening of the tendon sheath at the metacarpophalangeal joint often of the first finger of the right hand. The finger can be bent but not straightened without help.

Trigone. A triangle, *T. Vesicae.* Triangular space in the bladder, immediately behind the opening to the urethra.

Tri-iodothyronine. One of the thyriod hormones. Known as T^3 because its molecule contains 3 atoms of iodine.

Trinitrin. A name for nitro-glycerin, given in angina pectoris; it reduces blood pressure.

Triplegia. Paralysis of three limbs.

Triplets. Three children resulting from a single pregnancy. This occures about once in 7,800 labours.

Trismus. Lockjaw. Occurs as a reflex in dental caries. Is also a symptom of tetanus.

Trisomy. Division of chromosome 21 into three as in Down's syndrome.

Trocar. The perforating instrument used with a cannula to draw off fluids from the body.

Trochanter. Two processes (the greater and the lesser), at the juncture of the neck and shaft of femur.

Trochlear nerves. The fourth pair of cranial nerves. Motor nerves to the eyes.

Trophic. Relating to nutrition. Trophic ulcers occur where nutrition is poor, particularly if there is paralysis.

Trophoblast. The outer ectodermal layer of the embedding ovum.

Trousseau's sign. A spasm of the muscles occurring in tetany, if pressure is applied over large arteries or nerves.

Trunk. The torso.

Truss, An apparatus for retaining a hernia in place.

Trypanosoma, A genus of microscopic parasites which cause sleeping sickness and other diseases.

Trypanosomiasis, Infection with trypansomes.

Trypsin. The digestive enzyme of the pancreatic juice; acts on proteins.

Trupsinogen. A precursor of trypsin.

Tubegauz. Proprietary bandage of fine tubular cotton gauze made in many sizes from finger to body width. It is cool and light and does not ruck up.

Tubercle. (1) A small eminence. (2) The small greyish nodule which is the specific lesion of the tubercle bacillus.

Tuberculide. Any skin rash due to tuberculous infection.

Tuberculin. A preparation from cultures of the tubercle bacillus used in the diagnosis of tuberculosis. Many differnt tuberculins have been prepared in many (different ways, but new are) in common use. PPD is used for the intradermal. Mantoux tests, and for tuberculin patch test. Tuberculin PPD is also used for intradermal test. BCG vaccine is used for prophylaxis as an immunizing agent.

Tuberculoma. Walled-off region of caseating tuberculosis.

Tuberculosis. Infection with the Mycobacterium tuberculosis or tybercle bacillus. The human and bovine types attack man. Most infections enter by the respiratory tract and attack the lungs. Bovine bacilli, usually from infected milk, enter through the gastro intestinal tract, causing lesion in the tonsils, glands of neck, lining of the intestinal tract and mesenteric glands. The tubercle bacillus acts slowly and atiny nodule or tubercle forms in the affected area, which eventually calcifies. In most people, with good defences, no illness results from the primary infection and it probably serves to protect the patient against further attack. The person is termed *tuberculin positive* and this is ascertained by the Mantoux test (or other similar tests). BCG vaccination immunizes against tuberculosis by making a *tuberculin negative* person tuberculin positive. In a person who has contracted tuberculosis, the treatment is rest, good food and drug therapy, and the disease can be controlled, if diagnosed early, usually by x-ray.

Tuberculous. Connected with tuberculosis.

Tuberosity. Bony eminence.

Tuberous sclerosis. *See* EPILOIA.

Tubo- ovarian. Connected with both the Fallopian tube and the ovary (abscess, cyst,).

Tubule. Small tube.

Tularaemia. A disease transmitted to man from rabbits by blood sucking insect infected with B. tularense.

Tumerfaction. Becoming swollen.

Tumour. A swelling; an abnormal enlargement. Tumours may be *simple* or *malignant*; in the first case, they are not dangerous in themselves; in the second case, they are cancerous and produce secondary deposits in distant organs. Also they may be *solid* or *systic.*

Tunica. A term applied to several membranes, *e.g. T. vaginalis* the serous coat of the testicle.

Tuning fork. An instrument used for testing hearing. Each tuning fork bears a figure giving number of vibrations per second when it is struck, and a letter indicating the musical pitch (see RINNES TEST). It is also applied to the skin of other parts of the body to test the sense of vibration.

Turbinate bones. Tree thin convoluted bones situated on the lateral wall of each nasal fossa.

Turbinectomy. Operation to excise a turbinate bone.

Turgid. Swollen, distended.

Turner's syndrome. Ovarian agenesis. The patient is short in stature with webbed neck.

Tuissi. A cough.

Twin. One of two individuals born at one birth.

Tylosis. Thickening of the skin of the soles and palms.

Tympanites. A distended state of the abdomen caused by gas in the intestines.

Tympanitis. Otitis media.

Tympanoplasty, Operation to recon-struct the tympanum and the sound-conducting mechanism in middle ear.

Tympanum. Also called typanic cavity. A part of the middle ear, and comprises a cavity in the temporal bone deep to the typanic membrane. *T. membrane.* The membrane separating the middle from the external ear, commonly called the eardrum.

Typhlitis. Inflammation of the mucous surface of the caecum.

Typhoid Fever. An acute infections which flourishes where the standard of hygiene is poor. Caused by ingestion of the *Salmonella ryphi* from contaminated from contaminated food or water supplies. The germs reach the intestines and through the lymph channels produce a bacteraemia. After the first week the germs settle in the spleen, liver and intestines, especially the ileum. Here the lymph follicles known as Peyer's patches are attacked. They become inflamed, raised, and eventually the tissue of the follicle sloughs off. It is at this stage that intestinal haemorrhage or perforation may occur. Incubation period for the disease is 12–14 days and the patient remains infectious until bacteriological tests are negative. The onset is gradual. For 4 or 5 days the temperature is of the step-ladder type. If untreated, the patient becomes very ill during the second week with high temperature and slow pulse and the stools are often pea-soup in character. Rose-coloured spots, in crops, appear on the abdomen, chest and between the shoulder blades. By the third week, if untreated, the patient is delirious. The treatment is chloramphenicol, usually with dramatic improvement. *See also* ENTERIC FEVER.

Typhus fever. A highly infectious fever characerized by a petechial rash, high temperature and great prostration. It is caused by Rickettsia bodies from infected lice or rat fleas.

U

Ulcer. Means suppuration upon a surface. Ulcers can occur on skin or mucous membrane and may be acute or chronic.

Ulcerative. Pertaining to ulceration. *U. colitis.* A disease with inflammation and ulceration of the colon. There is diarrhoea, and mucus and blood are passed in the stools. The patient is anaemic.

Ulna. The inner bone of the forearm.

Ulnar. The name of an artery, a vein and a nerve running beside the ulna.

Ultrasonic. Of too high a frequency to be heard by the human ear.

Ultraviolet rays. Beyond the visible (seven colour) spectrum into which white light is resolved by a prism, there are non-visible rays (infra-red) at each end both below the red rays and above the violet rays (ultra-violet).

Umbilical cord. The funis; the cord connecting the fetus with the placenta.

Umbilicated. Having a navel-like depression, *e.g.* the papules in smallpox.

Umbilicus. Refers to a small depressed scar on the anterior abdominal wall. The navel.

Unciform. The hook shaped none of the wrist.

Uncinariasis. Infection with hookworm.

Unconsciousness. A state of not responding to stimuli, *e.g.* as a result of anaesthesia.

Undine, A thin glass flask with two spouts. Used for irrigation of eye.

Undulant. Wavelike. *U. fever. Malta fever.* A specific febrile disease. It is transmitted through cow's or goat's milk and runs a prolonged course.

Unguis. A fingernail.

Unna's paste. Treatment for ulcers of leg seldom used nowadays. It consists of zinc oxide, gelatin, glycerin and water. It is liquefied in a pot of hot water, and painted over a layer of gauze wrapped round the limb; if necessary a second coat may be applied and then the limb is surrounded by a thin bandage soaked in the mixture. When dry, it gives a thin plaster-like covering which keeps the part at rest.

Urachus. A fibrous cord in the fetus from the bladder to the umbilicus. It becomes the median umbilical ligament.

Uraemia. Accumulation of unknown toxic substances in the blood together with an increase in the blood urea and electrolyte imblance. It may be due to widespread renal disease or as a result of a greatly diminished fluid intake.

Uraemic fit. Epileptiform seizure resulting from a greatly raised blood urea.

Uraniscorrhaphy. Suture of a cleft plate.

Urea. One of the end-products of protein metabolism; the chief solid consitituent of urine. It is a diuretic.

Urea concentration test. The normal amount of urea in

urine is 2 per cent. If a definite quantity of urea, 15 grams in 100ml water, be given fasting—the amount of urea eliminated by the kidneys can be estimated by specimens taken 1, 2, and 3 hours after. The proper excretion of urea shows an adequately functioning kidney. the percentage should rise to 3 or 4. This test is used to estimate renal efficiency.

Uresis. Urination.

Ureter. The canal between the kidney and the bladder, down which the urine passes.

Ureteritis. Inflammation of a ureter.

Ureterocele. The result of congenital atresia of a ureteric orifice which causes a eystic enlargement of the portion of the ureter situated in the bladder wall.

Ureterolith. Stone in a ureter.

Ureterolithotomy. Operation for the removal of a stone impacted in the ureter.

Ureterosigmoidostomy. Implantation of a ureter into the sigmoid colon. The operation may be performed in cases of bladder disease.

Urethra. The canal between the bladder and the exterior through which the urine is discharged.

Urethritis. Inflammation of the urethra.

Urethrocele. Urethral diverticulum. A small pouch in the wall of the urethra more common in women than in men; the orgin is probably the result of a developmental defet.

Urethrography. X-ray examination of the urethra by means of retrograde injection of a radioopaque dy.

Urethroplasty. Plastic repair to the urethra.

Urethroscope. An instrument which si used for viewing the interior of the urethra.

Urethrotomy. Incision of the urethra to remedy stricture; the instrument used being a urethrotome.

Uric acid. Lithic acid; its presence in urine is discovered by its resemblance in colour to cayenne pepper. Frequently present gout. Liquor potassae dissolves this red deposit.

Urination. Micturition. The act of discharging urine.

Urine. The fluid secreted by the kidneys. The normal amount secreted in the twenty-four hours varies from 1 to $1\frac{1}{2}$ literes in an adult, 300 to 400ml in a child, 250 to 300ml in an infant. The normal constituents are water, salts, urea, acid bodies.

URINE TESTING

1. COLOUR: Normal, straw to light amber.

   (a) *Plate*. Low specific gravity urines are usually very pale.

   1. After drinking much fluid.
   2. In cold weather.
   3. Diabetes insipidus.
   4. Chronic nephritis.
   5. Diabetes mellitus (high specific gravity).

   (b) *High colour*. Concentrated urine.

   Concentration occurs:

   1. Reduced flud intake.
   2. Febrile disease, e.g. pneumonia, rheumatic fever.
   3. Profuse vomiting.
   4. Profuse diarrhoea.
   5. Profuse sweating.
   6. Heart disease.

   (c) *When coloured by blood it may be:*

   1. Bright red $\left.\rule{0pt}{18pt}\right\}$ If blood is present in large
   2. The colour of a dark beer $\quad$ amounts.
   3. Brownish if there is only a small amount of blood.

   (d) *When coloured by bile it may be:*

   Mahogany or greenish-brown, frothy.

2. QUANTITY: During 24 hours the normal output of urine is about 1500ml.

3. SPECIFIC GRAVITY of water is taken as 1.0 (formerly 1000).

   The SPECIFIC GRAVITY of water is taken as 1.0 (formerly 1000). The specific gravity of under depends on the amount of soluble solid matter, e.g. salts, urates, etc.

Normal specific gravity varies from 1-010 to 1-025.

Light-coloured urines, except in diabetes mellitus, as given in list under *colour*, are of low specific gravity and there is usually an increased ammount of urine passed.

Concentrated urines are of high specific gravity, and in diabetes mellitus may be 1-025 to 1-060.

with concentrated urine the quantity is usually decreased.

4. REACTION: Normal reaction-slightly acid, due to acid phosphates:

1. May be neutral.
2. May become alkaline:
   a. In cystitis.
   b. After taking alkalis.
   c. Specimen stale when tested.

5. SMELL: Normal, sweet.

In diabetes mellitus—very sweet, like new-mown hay.

In cystitis-ammoniacal, and often 'fishy'.

6. NAKED-EYE DEPOSITS:

1. *Urates*. Fawn, pink, or brick-red deposits occur in con-centrated urines when the urine becomes cold.
2. *Uric acid*. Small red grains, like cayenne pepper.
3. *Mucus*. Light flocculent deposit.
4. *Pus*. Thick yellow or greenish-yellow.
5. *Blood*. Clots or brownish deposit.
6. *Phosphates*. Thick white deposit.

To test a specimen of urine

1. Note the colour.
2. Note the specific gravity.
3. Note the reaction. This is tested with blue or red lit-

mus paper.

    a. Blue litmus turns red = acid reaction.

    b. Red litmus turns blue = alkaline reaction.

    c. Red and blue litmus do not change = neutral.

4. Note the smell.

5. Note the naked-eye deposits.

    In many cases a bacteriological examination of the urine isrequired.

Tests for albumin

(a) *Albustix Reagent Strips*

Proceed according to instructions on bottle.

Tests (b) or (c) may be carried out if Albustix is not available.

(b) *Heat*

1. Fill $\frac{2}{3}$ test tube with urine.

2. If not acid, add 2 or 3 drops of acetic acid.

3. Heat the upper $\frac{1}{3}$ of the urine until it boils.

4. The part heated becomes white and opaque.

5. Add 2 or 3 drops of acetic acid.

    a. The deposit remains = albumin.

    b. The deposit clears up = phosphates.

A cloudy urine which becomes clear on heating = urates.

(c) *Salicyl-sulphonic acid*

Take 10 drops of urine in a test tube. If alkaline, add 3 drops of acetic acid. Add 1 drop of salicyl-sulphonic acid 25%. If a cloud forms albumin is present.

(d) *Estimation of quantity of albumin by an Esbach's albuminometer.*

Render the urine acid if not already so.

If the specific gravity is higher than 1·010 dilute with an equal quantity of water.

Take a graduated Esbach's tube and put in rine up to the mark U. Add Esbach's solution up to mark R. Cork tube and mix by carefully inverting. Carefully label tube with patient's name and date and time. Let it stand for twenty-four hours. Read off the height of deposit in tube and record as grams per litre.

If the urine was diluted, the result must multiplied by 2.

Tests for blood

(a) *Occultest Reagent Tablets*

Proceed according to instructions on bottle.

Test (b) may be carried out if Occultest tablets are not available.

(b) *Tincture of guaiacum and ozonic ether*

1. Stir the specimen.
2. Pour about 5ml of urine into a test tube.
3. Add 2 drops of tincture of guaiacum.
4. Shake and mix.
5. Add slowly 3 to 4 ml of ozonic ether.

A blue ring appears at the junction of the fluids when blood is present. (A similar result is obtained if a patient is taking potassium iodide.)

Tests for sugar

(a) *Clinitest Reagent Tablets*

This is a test for all sugars. Proceed according to instructions on bottle.

(b) *Clinistix Reagent Strips*

This is a test for glucose only. Proceed according to instructions on bottle.

(c) *Benedict's test*

This test is only carried out if Clinitest tablets are not available.

1. Take 5ml of Benedict's solution and to this add 8 drops of urine with a pipette.

2. Boil for three minutes.

If sugar is present the colour will change. Greenish-yellow denotes a trace of sugar; yellow: some sugar; and orange-brown: much sugar.

Tests for acetone

(a) *Acetest Reagent Tablets*

Proceed according to instructions on bottle.

(b) *Rothera's test*

This test is only carried out if Acetest tablets are not available.

1. To half a test tube full of urine add ammonium sulphate crystals until the liquid is saturated.

2. Dissolve two or three nitro-prusside crystals in 8ml of water and add four drops of this to the urine.

3. Shake well.

4. Add ten drops of strong ammonia.

There will be a purple colour in 15 minutes if acetone or diacetic acid is present.

Tests for bilirubin

(a) *Ictotest Reagent Tablets*

Proceed according to instructions on bottle.

(b) *Iodine test*

This test in only used if Ictotest tablets are not available. To 5ml of urine add a few drops of tincture of iodine which has been diluted with equal parts of water.

A green ring will form where the two liquids join if bilirubin is present.

Special reagent strips may be available which give a combined test for a number of abnormalities in the urine. The given procedure should be followed meticulously, particularly the timing of the reading of results.

Any nurse who knows that she is colourblind should have her tests checked.

Uriniferous tubules. Numerous minute tubules in the kindey which secrete urine.

Urinometer. A small glass instrument with a graduated stem. It is used for measuring the specific gravity of urine.

Urobilin. One of the pigments of the urine, derived from bile pigments.

Urobilinogen. Derivative of bilirubin which is made in the intestine by the gut bacteria. Some of it is absorbed and, in circumstances in which there is impaired liver function, may be excreted in the urine.

Urochrome. Pigment colouring urine.

Urography. X-ray of the urinary tract.

Urokinase. Enzyme found in the urine. In disease states it can cause bleeding from the kindey.

Urolith. A stone found in the urine.

Urologist. A specialist in urology.

Urology. Refers to the study of diseases of the urinary tract.

Uroscopy. Examination of the urine.

Uterogestation. The period of pregnancy.

Uterovesical. Relating to the uterus and the bladder.

Uterus. Womb. Muscular hollow pelvic organ. In the resting state it measures about 7.5 × 5cm and is triangular in shape with a cervix about 2-5cm which projects into the vagina. It is connected bilaterally to the oviducts (Fallopian tubes). The uterus has a glandular epithelium lining it and the whole structure is under the control of sex hormones, in particular oestrogens and progesterone. See MENSTRUATION. The uterus is the normal site of implantation of the trophoblast. During pregnancy the uterus grows out of the pelvis to occupy much of the abdominal cavity.

Utricle. (1) The larger sac of membrane in the vestibule of the internal ear. (2) The prostatic vesicle.

Uvea, uveal tract. The middle coat of the eyeball. The choroid, ciliary body and iris as a whole.

Uveitis. Inflammation of the uvea.

Uvula. A small fleshy body hanging down at the back of the soft palate.

Uvulectomy. Excision of uvula.

Uvulitis. Inflammation of the uvula.

Vaccination. (1) Inoculation of cow-poxlymph into the arm as a protection from smallpox. (2) Protective inoculation with any vaccine.

Vaccine. An extract or suspension of attenuated or killed organisms. The antigenic properties of the organism are retained and the vaccine is used to immunize the recipient.

Vaccinia. Cowpox. In man, it gives immunity to smallpox and therefore used in vaccination against that disease.

Vagina. The passage leading from the cervix uteri to the vulva. The lower limit of this canal is the hymen.

Vaginismus. Spasmodic contraction of vagina whenever the vulva or vagina is touched.

Vaginitis. Inflammation of the vagina.

Vagotomy. Surgical division of the vagus nerve sometimes performed on patients with peptic or duodenal ulcers.

Vagus. The pneumogastric nerve.

Valvotomy. Incision into a valve, especially heart valve. The purpose of the operaton is to widen the orific of a stenosed valve.

Valvulae conniventes. transverse folds of mucous membrane in the upper part of the small intestine.

Van den Bergh's test. Performed to discover the presence of bile pigment in the blood. It also differentiates between the pigment retained in the blood from obstruction of the bile passages, and that due to haemolysis.

Varicocele. A varicose condition of the veins of the spermatic cord.

Varicose ulcer. Ulceration of the lower legs due to reduction in the blood supply resulting from increased venous pressure.

Varicose veins. Dilated veins in which the valves have become incompetent. As a result the blood flow may become reversed or static. Most common in the legs where the blood pools by gravitation. Other examples are piles and oesophageal varices.

Varicotomy. Excision of varicose vein.

Varioloid. A mild form of smallpox, sometimes seen in persons who have been previously vaccinated.

Varix. An enlarged and tortuous vein.

Vas. A vessel, or duct of the body; as vas deferens, the duct of the testis.

Vascular. Possesing many blood vessels.

Vascular system. System of blood vessels.

Vasectomy. Removal of a part of the vas deferens.

Vasoconstriction. Contraction of blood vessels.

Vasodilatation. Dilatation of blood vessels.

Vasomotor. Concerned with constriction of blood vessels. *V. nerves.* Sympathetic nerves which control the tone of smooth muscle in the walls of blood vessels.

Vasospasm. Spasm of the blood vessels.

Vasovagal syndrome. Slowing of the heart rate with a feeling of nausea and grave distress. The attack may last a few minutes or an hour. The cause is unknown.

vater's ampulla. Small dilation in the terminal portion of the common bile duct where it empties into the duodenum.

Vector. A carrier. One who conveys the infection to another person.

Vena cava. The superior vena cava and the inferior vena cava are two large veins which return blood from the head and body and empty it into the right atrium of the heart.

Venepuncture. Inserting a needle into a vein.

Venereal. Relating to sexual intercourse. *V. disease.* Infectious diseases transmitted during sexual intercourse. *e.g.* genorrhoea, syphilis.

Venereology. The study of venereal disease.

Venesection. Blood-letting. A vein is opened and blood drained off from it. Frequently performed in the past for almost any ailment. There are very few present-day indications for venesection.

Venography. X-ray examination of veins following injection of contrast medium.

Ventricles. The two lower chambers of the heart are known as the right and left ventricles. The cavities in the brain also are known as ventricles.

Ventriculography. X-ray examination of the ventricles of the brain. Air or a radio-opaque dye is introduced into the ventricles, enabling their size and position to be observed.

Ventrofixation. The operation to suture an abdominal viscus to the anterior abdominal wall.

Ventrosuspension. Another operation having the same object as ventrofixation, but fixing the round ligaments instead of the uterus to the abdominal wall.

Venule. Small vein.

Vermicide. Substance able to kill worms in the intestine.

Vermifuge. Substance used to dispel worms.

Verminous. Infested with animal parasites.

Vernix caseosa. The sebaceous material which covers the skin of the fetus.

Version. The operation of altering the presentation of the fetus in the uterus so as to facilitate its delivery. *Cephalic version* is turning the fetus, so that the head peresents, while podalic version brings about a breech presentation. *Bipolar version*, version by acting upon both poles of the fetus.

Vertebrae. The thirty-three small bones which form the backbone, or spinal column.

Vertex. The crown of the head.

Vertigo. Giddiness.

Vesica. The bladder.

Vesical. Relating to the bladder.

Vesicant. A blistering agent.

Vesicle. A blister. Blisters of greater diameter than 5mm are termed bullae. Blisters contain serum.

Vesicovaginal. Relating to the bladder and the vagina.

Vesicular breathing. The normal sound of inspiration heard on auscultation.

Vesiculitis. Inflammation of seminal vesicles.

Vestibular neuronitis. Disorder affecting the vestibular nerve which is characterized by extreme vertigo while hearing is unaffected. May result from streptomycin toxicity.

Vestibule. A small cavity of the ear into the which the cochlea opens. (2) The space between the labia minora.

Vestigial. Rudimentary. Bearing a trace of something now vanished or degenerate.

Vibrio. A genus of micro-organisms shaped like a bacillus but curved. One causes cholera.

Vicarious. When one organ performs the work of another. *V. menstruation.* Menstruation from a passage other than the uterus.

Villi. Fine soft processes of living cells. *Intestinal v.* in the small intestines each contain a central vessel or lacteal, surrounded by a plexus of capillaries. Their function is to increase the surface area of the small intestine thereby aiding absorption. *Chorionic v.* Processes arising from the chorion, the outer membrane of the developing ovum. Specialization of a mass of villi ultimately forms the placenta.

Villous. Having the nature of villi, thus a villous tumour of the bladder is a growth consisting of long slender processes of cells.

Vincent's angina. Infection of the mucous epithelium of the mouth by a symbiotic (*see symbiosis*) association of a spirochaete Borrelia vincenti and a fusiform Gramnegative bacsterium Fusobacterium planti-vincenti.

Vinegar. A weak solution of acetic acid formed by fermentation of wine and other alcoholic liquids.

Viraemia. Viruses present in the blood stream.

Virilism. The appearance of masculine characteristics in the female.

Virology. The study of viruses and the diseases caused by them.

Virus. Infecting agent that will pass through the finest filter known. *e.g.* the cause of mumps, anterior poliomyelitis and other infectious diseases.

Viscera. The internal organs of the great cavities of the body, the term being generally applied to the abdomen, *Sing. viscus.*

Visceroptosis. Prolapse of the abdominal viscera.

Viscopaste. Proprietary zinc paste bandage.

Vision. The act or faculty of seeing. *Binocular vision,* use of both eyes without seeing double. *Central vision, direct vision* that performed through the centre of the retina. *Double vision, diplopia,* a failure to fuse the images thrown upon the two restinae at the same time: two images are therefore seen and object appear double. May be due to defect in muscles of the eye or an error of refraction. It is also a symptom of some nervous diseases, *e.g,* encephalitis lethargica. *Peripheral vision, indirect vision,* that performed by the peripheral or circumferential portion of the retina. *Stereoscopic vision,* that which gives perception of distance and solidity.

Vitallium. an alloy used in bone surgery for nails, screws, plates, etc.

Vitamins. Chemical substances present in food, necessary for health and development. Those at present known are:

A. anti-infective, fat soluble; found in animal fat such a butter, cream, milk, fish oil and derived from carotin, the colouring matter of carrots and tomatoes. Lack of A causes a lowered resistance to infection, night blindness and opacity of the cornea

B. Compelx (has different parts). Water soluble, found in whole- meal cereals, yeast, Mcarmite, liver, lean meat. B^1, or thiamine, anti-neuritic; prevents polyneuritis and beriberi B^2, or riboflavin; deficiency causes a syndrome which includes visual disturbances. B^6, or pyridoxine: no deficiency symptoms are known, but the drug has been used in irradiation and pregnancy sickness. B^{12}, or cyanocobalamin, the specific anti-anaemia principle of liver. Nicotinic acid is also a constituent of the B complex.

C. Anti-scorbutic; found in rose hips, black currants oranges, tomatoes, raw vegetables. Lack of C causes scurvy.

D. Anit-rachitic; found in animal fats and fish oils. The action of ultraviolet rays on certain fats, known as sterols produces vitamin D. It is necessary for the metabolism of calcium. Lack of vitamin D causes rickets.

E. Anit-sterility; found in wheat germ oil, an ingrdient of whole wheat. Lack of E causes sterility and insecurity of pregnancy.

K. The 'Koagulation Vitamin'. Fat soluble. Occurs in the green part of plants particularly, alfala, grass, spinach, kale, carrot tops and vegetable oils. It may be formed by bacterial action from food in the lower part of the intestine and absorbed. Bile salts in the intestine are necessary for absorpation. Lack of vitamin K causes a deficiency of prothrombin in the blood, which is necessary for the clotting of blood. Prescribed in cases of obstructive jaundice.

Vitiligo. Disorder of pigment cells in which patches of depigmented skin arise, often in a symmetrical distribution.

Vitreous chamber of the eye. The posterior five-sixths of the eyeball, that part behind the lens. It is filled with a clear jelly-like substance called the *vitreous humour.*

Vitriol. Any crystalline sulphate. Blue vitriol copper sulphate or blue stone. Sometimes applied to granulation tissue on the eyelids. *Oil of v.* Sulpuric acid.

Vivisection. Scientific examination of living animal.

Vocal cords. Two folds of mucous membrane in the larynx attached behind to the arytenoid cartilages, and in front to the back of the thyroid cartilage. Voice is produced by variation in position ofthese cords when acted on by small muscles of the larynx, and at the same time forcing through them an expiratory blast of air.

Volatile. That which evaporates quickly.

Volition. The act or power of willing.

Volkmann's paralysis V. contracture. A muscular paralysis caused by applying splints too tighty so that the blood supply is impaired. Most commonly seen in the forearm after fractures about the elbow joint.

Volkmann's spoon. A sharp spoon used for scraping a septic cavity.

Volvulus. A twisting of a piece of intestine of its mesenteric attachment. Acute intestinal obstruction is the result.

Vomer. A bone of the septum of the nose.

Vomit, To eject the contents of the stomach through the mouth. Projectile V. Forcible ejection of gastric contents without warning.

Vomiting of pregnancy. The vomiting to which about two-thirds of pregnant women are subject at some time or other during the period of gestation. Occures usually about the second third and forth months, and is commonest in the morning. In most cases no ill results follow, but occasionally the vomiting becomes so frequent and severe that a grave condition is produced, called the *intractable*, or *pernicious vomiting ofpregnancy*, or *hyperemesis* gravidarum. Vomiting is also a symptom of toxaemia of pregnancy.

Von Gierke's disease. Glycogen storage disease. Recessively inherited defect in the metabolism of glycogen so that it cannot be used. The tissues become stuffed with glycogen while hypoglycaemia occurs.

Von Reckling hausen's disease. Characterized by multiple tumours along cutaneous nerves of trunk and scalp, with areas of pigment ation.

Vulsellum. Catch forceps with toothed blades.

Vulva. The external organs of generation of the female.

Vulvectomy. Excision of vulva.

Vulvitis. Inflammation of the vulva.

Vulvovaginal. Pertaining to the vulva and the vagina.

Vulvovaginitis. Inflammation of both the vulva and the vagina.

W

Waldeyer's ring. Circle of adenoid tissue in the pharynx formed by the faucial, lingual and pharyngeal tonsils.

Wallerian degeneration. Degeneration of a nerve after it has been cut or severed.

Wart. Small horny tumour from the skin. The *common wart* is due to a virus infection. A *plantar wart* is found on the sole of the foot. *Venereal warts* are common warts on the genitalia and not to be confused with flat condylomata of secondary syphilis.

Wassermann reaction. A blood test which shows whether the individual from whome the blood is taken is or is not subject of active syphilis. Sometimes the cerebrospinal fluid is taken instead of blood.

Water beds. Rubber mattress filled with warm water and used to prevent pressure sores.

Water-brash. Regurgitation of stomach acid into the oesophagus and thence to the mouth.

Waterhouse Friderichsen syndrome. Syndrome resulting from bilateral adrenal haemorrhage accompanying the purpura of acute septicaemia, usually meningococcal.

Weal. A white or pinkish elevation on the skin, as in urticaria.

Wean. To cease feeding a baby at the breast.

Weber syndrome. Hemianopia caused by posterior cerebral aneurysm.

Weil's disese. Epidemic spirochaetal jaundice. Disease caused by a Leptospira characterized by fever headache, and pains in the limbs. Many patients develop jaundice and a purpuric rash.

Weil Felix reaction, An agglutination reaction for typhus.

Welch's bacillus. Clostridium perfringens, a sporen-forming organism found in gas gangrene.

Wernicke's. Encephalopathy. Syndrome occurring in association with alcoholic polyneuritis, characterized by vertigo, nystagmus, ataxia and stupor. Considered to be due to thiamine deficiency.

Wertheim's operation. A radical operation for uterine cancer, where- by the uterus, tubes, ovaries, broad ligaments, pelvic lymph nodes and cellular tissue around ureters are removed en masse.

Wharton's duct. The duct of the submaxillary gland.

Wharton's jelly. A special tissue of the umbilical cord.

Wheelhouse's operation. External (perineal) urethrotomy for stricture of the urethra.

Whey. The liquid left after milk has been clotted with rennin.

Whipple's disease. Intestinal lipodystrophy. Disease of unknown cause. There is progressive deposition of mucoprotein material in the wall of the small intestine.

Whites. A popular term for leucorrhoea.

Whitfield's ointment. Contains salicylic and benzoic acids. Used for athlete's foot and ringworm.

Whitlow, Inflammation near a finger-nail, with suppuration.

See ONYCHIA.

Whooping cough. Pertussis.

Widal reaction. A blood test for typhoid fever. Not available until patient has been ill for about ten days.

Willebrand's disease. Inherited defect of blood vessels and clotting mechanism.

Wilms' tumour. A ongenital tumour of the kidney which is malignant.

Wilson's disease. A rare metabolic disorder (hepatolenticular degeneration) in which copper accumulates in the liver and certain nuclei of the brain.

Windpipe. The trachea.

Winslow's foramen. An aperture between the stomach and liver formed by folds of peritoneum. It forms a communication between the greater and lesser peritoneal cavities.

Wisdom teeth. The posterior molars. They erupt last, usually when a person is about 21 years old.

Womb. The uterus.

Wood's glass. Glass which contains nickel oxide. It causes fluorescence of certain objects and is used to detect ringwrom. —

Worm. Invertebrate animal.

Wound. Injury.

Wrist. The joint between the hand and the forearm. The carpus.

Writer's cramp. Spasm of the hand and forearm brought on by efforts to write. largely due to defective posture when writing.

X

X chromosome. The sex chromosome which is paired in the homogametic sex. Unlike the Y chromosome it carries many major genes.

Xanthelasma. A condition in which yellow patches or nodules occur on the skin especially in the eyelids.

Xanthine. A nitrogenous substance produced in the body. Sometimes found in the urine.

Xanthochromia. The distinctive yellow colour of cerebrospinal fluid following a subarachnoid haemorrhage. It is due to haemolysis of the blood in the subarachnoid space, and indicates that subarachnoid heamorrhage has occurred.

Xanthoderma. Yellowness of the skin.

Xanthoma. The same as xanthelasma.

Xenopsylla cheopis. A rat flea which can transmit plague and typhus.

Xenopus test. Test for pregnancy. The mother's urine is injected into the lymph sac of a female toad. If the woman is pregnant, the toad will pass ova, in from 24-48 hours. Now obsolete.

Xeroderma. A dry state of the skin.

Xeropthalmia. Ulceration of the cornea occurring in

vitamin A deficiency.

Xeroradiography. The technique for soft tissue radiography using special equipment giving a positive print.

Xerosis. Abnormal dryness, *e.g.* of the conjunctiva or the skin.

Xerostomia. Dryness of the mouth.

Xiphoid process. A sword-shaped cartilage attached to the breast bone. Also called the ensiform cartilage.

Y

Y chromosome. Sex chromosome found only in the heterogametic sex (male). It is shorter than the X chromosome and usually carries few major genes.

Yaws. Framboesis. Tropical disease, resembling syphilis, caused by treponema pertenue.

Yeast, Unicellular fungi, ascomycetes, which possess enzymes capable of converting sugars into ethanol with the release of carbone dionide. Yeasts are also used as sources of protein and vitamins.

Yellow fever. Virus-mediated diease transmitted by mosquitoes. Characterized by fever, prostratiseon jaundice and gastro- intestinal haemorrhage.

Ziehil- Neelsen's stain. Staining technique used to identify tubercle bacilli by their ability to retain the stain when treated with acid; hence acid-fast bacilli.

Zinc. A metallic element. The chloride is used as a caustic and disinfectant. Zinc oxide ointment is used for dressing mionr ulceration of the skin.

Zollinger-Ellison syndrome. Increased production of acid gastric juice in response to gastrin secreted by pancreatic neoplasm, resulting in peptic ulceration and inactivation of enzymes of small intestine which operate only in the alkaline range.

Zondek-Aschheim test. To diagnose pregnancy. The urine of a pregnant woman contains a counterpart of the luteinizing hormone of the pituitary gland where the diagnosis is uncertain, the urine is injected into immature mice. A few days later the mice are killed and if the generative organs of the mice have undergone the changes characteristic of puberty the woman is known to be pregnant.

Zonula ciliaris. Suspensory ligament of lens of the eye.

Zoogloea layer. Colonies of bacteria in a jelly-like layer. Found on the top of a sand filter bed. This layer contains algae and protozoa and helps in water purification.

Zoosperm. Same as spermatozoon.

Zoster. Shingles.

Zygoma. The cheekbone.

Zygote. The cell formed, by combination of ovum with spermalazoon.

Zymotic. A term which includes all epidemic endemic and contagious diseases arising from germs.